# POSITIVE SOBRIETY

## A Comprehensive, Integrative, and Evidence-Based Approach to Addiction Treatment

*Daniel H. Angres M.D.*

Copyright © 2012, Revised 2015

Daniel H. Angres, MD
All Rights Reserved.

ISBN-10: 1480179167
ISBN-13: 9781480179165

CreateSpace Independent Publishing Platform,
North Charleston, South Carolina

This book is dedicated to:

Kathy Bettinardi-Angres, my wife and partner in establishing our program nearly three decades ago. Kathy was not only critical in the establishment of this program and the design described in this manual but in its development and maintenance. Without her insight, clinical and administrative skills, this program and design would not be in existence. I also dedicate this book to our two children, Dominic and Rachel.

and…

*To our patients, past, present, and future*

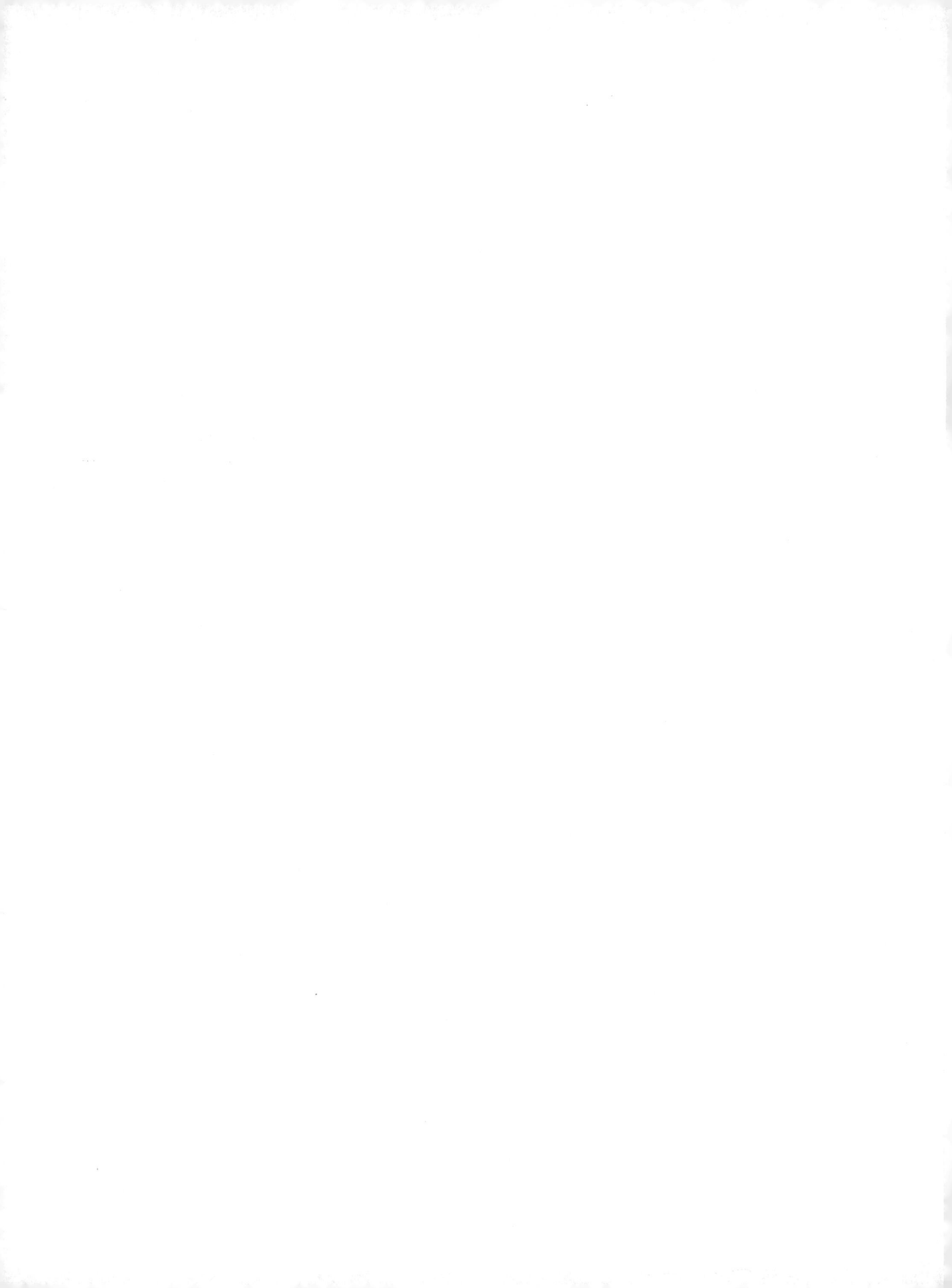

# Contents:

Acknowledgments ........................................................................................................... 9
Preface ............................................................................................................................ 11

1) What is Positive Sobriety? ........................................................................................ 13

2) Understanding the Disease of Addiction ................................................................. 17
    Reward ..................................................................................................................... 22
    Learning and Memory ............................................................................................ 24
    Motivation ............................................................................................................... 25
    Decision Making ..................................................................................................... 27
    Behavioral Addictions and Addictive Interactive Disorders ................................ 29
    Nicotine Dependence ............................................................................................. 31
    Hardware Problems and Hardware Solutions ...................................................... 33
    Hardware Treatment Interventions ....................................................................... 34
    Specific Medications for Addiction and Comorbid Issues ................................... 35
    Chronic Pain ........................................................................................................... 37

3) Psychosocial Treatment: Software Treatment Interventions ................................. 41
    Our Treatment Structure ....................................................................................... 42
    A) Individualized Treatment Planning and Individual Therapy ......................... 44
    B) Small Group Therapy ........................................................................................ 46
    C) Therapeutic Community ................................................................................... 49
    D) Family Program ................................................................................................. 50
    E) Twelve-Step Programs ....................................................................................... 52
    F) Volunteerism ...................................................................................................... 54
    G) Diet and Exercise .............................................................................................. 56
    H) Continuing Care ................................................................................................ 59

## 4) Core Treatment Lectures and Workshops ... 61
- Denial ... 61
- Grief ... 62
- Anger ... 64
- Post-Acute Withdrawal Syndrome (PAWS) ... 69
- Relapse ... 70
- AA: 1 and 2 ... 71
- Shame and Guilt ... 72
- Codependency ... 74
- Common Symptoms of Codependency ... 75
- Impact of Addiction on Loved Ones ... 77
- Stages of Change ... 78
- Trauma and Recovery ... 81

## 5) Who Are You? Personality and Addiction ... 85
- Self, No Self ... 85
- Narcissism, Addictive Personality, and Quantum Change ... 86
- The Millon ... 94

## 6) What Are You Looking For? ... 97
- Early and Longer-Term Recovery ... 98
- Other Ways to Find What You Are Looking For ... 102

## 7) What Makes You Happy? ... 105
- 1) Self-Acceptance, Taking Responsibility ... 107
- 2) Cultivating Optimism and Gratitude ... 108
- 3) Goals that support a senses of Meaning and Purpose ... 108
- 4) Forgiveness ... 110
- 5) Kindness ... 110
- 6) Increased Connection with Family and Friends ... 111
- 7) Mindfulness ... 112
- 8) Doing the Next Right Thing ... 112
- 9) Flow ... 114
- 10) Spirituality ... 114

8) Developing a Meditation Practice ................................................................................117
   Meditation: The Antidote to Hedonic Adaptation ..............................................117
   Meditative Aids and Approaches .........................................................................122
   Two Guided Meditations......................................................................................126

9) Positive Sobriety Worksheets ........................................................................................131
   Who Are You? Personality and Addiction ..........................................................131
   What Are You Looking For?................................................................................134
   What Makes You Happy? ....................................................................................138

References ..........................................................................................................................155

# Acknowledgments

There have been many clinicians past and present who have contributed to the evolution of this program and design and who have implemented the program to the benefit of so many patients. Some of these clinicians are mentioned under core treatment lectures that they helped develop.

There was considerable editorial assistance from Jessica Kryzkowski, PsyD, who also provided content about individual therapy and use of the Millon.

Phillip Chow has of great assistance in helping explain and implement the Big Five personality inventory.

Stephanie Bologeorges assisted in edits and contributions throughout the book, organizing the references, including some in-text and research components in the appendix, and developing the extensive resource section.

A special thank-you to Cindy Power, who helped us set up the AID component of the program, and Mona Villarreal, who has transformed the yoga experience for our patients.

I also thank the many alumni, volunteers, and students who contributed to the evolution of this manuscript in their own unique ways. And finally to Paul Feldman, MD (1950–2007), and his many contributions to our program and patients. You will always be remembered.

# Preface

Addiction can be understood as an extreme form of attachment, one that creates an exaggeration of the human condition—a condition in which we are prone to look outside of ourselves for well-being. The exaggeration exists in addicts because we are biogenetically and otherwise predisposed to the power of the addictive process. This book will examine a way out of this attachment that can both promote abstinence and transform the pain and suffering of addiction into a path to greater well-being and happiness.

The recovering addict seeks happiness like anyone else. The failure to work a program of recovery can mean more than just unhappiness; it can mean relapse. Since addiction is a chronic and progressive disease, continued relapse can mean severe disability and even death, so staying sober is imperative.

The disease of addiction will always be present even if it is quiescent during long-term recovery. An AA member once warned me to never become overconfident in recovery. He said the disease is always there; "doing push-ups and ready to pounce". This situation can facilitate a strong program of recovery. The recovering addict's life depends on consistent efforts to minimize the effects of this chronic process. Reminiscent of the constant irritation that creates a pearl in some oysters, this disease can lay the foundation of happiness and well-being in recovering addicts.

The various aspects of this path as outlined in this book have served many of us well. This book presents a comprehensive approach that integrates many evidence-based strategies that have been noted to facilitate recovery and well-being. The abstinence-based, twelve-step-oriented treatment approach (the Minnesota Model) has been in existence since the early 1940s, shortly after the creation of Alcoholics Anonymous in 1935. I have personally benefited from this model, as it directly contributed to what is at this writing, thirty-two years of sobriety. For the past thirty years, I have been able to develop a program for addicted professionals now housed with the Positive Sobriety Institute in Chicago, Illinois. With a skilled and dedicated staff, we have been able to facilitate recovery for thousands of addicted patients. We have learned many things about treatment over the years. This includes the importance of moving beyond abstinence and into optimal well-being. Happiness and well-being will assist in the maintenance of sobriety, just as sobriety will assist in the maintenance of happiness.

Chapter 1 discusses the latest findings of the positive psychology movement and how it relates to addiction. Chapter 2 outlines what we know about the neurobiology of addiction. Chapters 3 and 4 walk through the treatment components we use in our addiction setting. Chapter 5 explores the interface of personality and addiction, chapter 6 explores motivations for use, and Chapter 7 explores the elements of happiness. Chapter 8 looks at developing a meditation practice, and Chapter 9 provides worksheets to assist in putting these concepts into operation. The appendix includes links to helpful resources.

This book will serve different purposes. If you are in our Positive Sobriety Institute Program, it will serve as a guide and resource as you progress through the program to aftercare and beyond. If you are not in our program, it can walk you through this program. This book is not meant as a substitute for a treatment program, but it will present alternatives to those who are not in a program for whatever reason. Perhaps it can direct those in need to where they need to go for their recovery.

There is a substantial amount of scientific detail in some sections. You may want all, some, or none of this detail. There is a summary section called "Plainly Stated" in bold after some of these sections for those who want to cut to the chase.

You will also see a section called "Alternative Option" at the end of selected sections of the book that will guide the reader not in a program. Additionally, several sections will also include a "Personal Perspective." This perspective will draw on my experiences in treatment and recovery and hopefully will add a more intimate look at some of what is discussed.

You will have the opportunity to take self-reports that can inform you of areas of individual strengths and weaknesses. This allows for ongoing self-evaluation. There are also ways to identify various motivations for use. This book emphasizes the benefits of twelve-step recovery and describes how the field of positive psychology is aligned with this recovery model. The combined effect of abstinence and character development can create something positive out of a negative. I call this ongoing effort "positive sobriety." I hope this manual and workbook assist you in this effort.

— *Daniel H. Angres, MD*

# 1. What Is Positive Sobriety?

The *American Heritage Dictionary*, 2nd edition, defines "sobriety" as "seriousness or gravity; solemnity" as well as "absence of alcoholic intoxication." This would make "positive sobriety" seem like an oxymoron. No doubt, abstinence in addiction requires serious effort. Certainly, the initiation of a program of abstinence is typically a solemn affair. However, the first promise of Alcoholics Anonymous, "We came to know a new freedom and new happiness" (1976) speaks to better things to come. The concept of positive sobriety is dedicated to the idea that recovery from addiction is a combination of solemn effort and pursuit of happiness.

Over the past few decades, serious effort has been made to better understand what brings people happiness and how to better access it. Research suggests that what we commonly think will bring us happiness, such as money, beauty, or fame, will only temporarily succeed. Something called "hedonic adaptation," that is, getting used to pleasurable experiences, will eventually intercede (Brickman and Campbell 1971). People get used to pleasurable experiences just like they get used to unpleasant ones and this ability to adapt can be both protective and dampening. Pursuing elusive goals such as money, beauty, and fame brings temporary pleasure or happiness at best. Pursuing repeated pleasure (or absence of pain) in addiction is beyond elusive; it's dangerous. The continued use of mood-altering substances and behaviors (food, sex, gambling) despite adverse consequences underscores just how dangerous addiction is.

What is so fascinating about the current research on happiness is that it contends that people often deceive themselves about what really will make them happy. This, of course, is cultivated by our culture, especially through the media, that the next thing consumed will give one a sense of sustained well-being. Just looking at all the happy faces on commercials for beer, fast-food restaurants, hair products, and the like demonstrates how this is cultivated in the current culture. This often-shared illusion keeps people in a state of chronic frustration and deprivation, as the media tactics only offer empty promises. Any relative gains in feelings of happiness that come from consumption quickly abate.

Dr. Ben-Shahar, in his 2007 book *Happier*, described happiness as ultimately being a balance between pleasure and meaning. Pleasure is involved with present benefit, and meaning with future benefit. Long-term sustained happiness is a combination of these two. So, if one has a certain goal that has a sense of purpose and meaning and that goal is congruent with who one is (what is sometimes described as "self-concordant"), then the person should be able to enjoy the pursuit as well as the attainment of that goal. In fact, enjoying the effort in pursuing a given meaningful goal becomes more important and potentially more rewarding than the actual attainment of it. The path of recovery (and happiness) requires a persistent effort in balancing present benefit with future benefit, and at times sacrificing pleasure for meaning. The key is learning how to enjoy the journey. This comes from knowing yourself and making sure your goals are self-concordant, that is, that you follow a path because it is what you want for yourself, not because it is expected of you. This purposeful action is reflective of the idea of recovery coming from within. The importance of self-concordance will be explored throughout this book.

Specialists in the addiction field are learning from the relatively new field of positive psychology. Their research confirms what was suspected all along: age, race, income (above the poverty line), success, and even physical illness do not ultimately determine well-being. Cloninger (1994) described three essential elements along the path to well-being: letting go, working in the service of others, and growing in self-awareness. Sonja Lyubomirsky, PhD, in *The How of Happiness* (2008), outlined what brings true happiness or well-being, as demonstrated by research. This includes forgiving, practicing optimism, being connected and kind to others, and having spirituality. Lyubomirsky also demonstrated that while 50 percent of our happiness is determined by genetics and another 10 percent by our circumstances, 40 percent is available for our own efforts in this pursuit. You may recognize the parallels in percentages between Lyubomirsky's happiness components and Dick and Beirut's (2006) discussion of the genetic factors of addiction described later.

It is possible to learn ways to cultivate and practice these proven paths to happiness and well-being. The work of early sobriety is hard, indeed solemn. Things often need to get worse before they get better. But getting back to baseline will not be enough to maintain long-term sobriety. In fact, abstinence without well-being is referred to as being a "dry drunk". Addicts need true happiness like anyone else. The well-being therapies promoted in this text have demonstrated reduced dropout rates and relapses in anxiety states and depression (Hubbard 1997), and are demonstrating similar effects in the recovery from addiction. The program elements described in this book, including therapy, lectures, meditation, investment in twelve-step recovery, and family therapy, are designed to assist you in this journey toward a positive sobriety. One cannot invest only in abstinence; one must also do the work involved in the pursuit of true happiness in sobriety.

The struggle for the addict is to first and foremost know they are on a hedonic treadmill chasing an increasingly elusive high. The addict loses perspective of this fact because of denial, the close companion of addiction, and feeds off the progressive deterioration of what makes us uniquely human: the ability to freely choose. Denial is reinforced by both the powerful reward of the addiction and the deficits in learning, motivation, memory, and decision making that accompany the process. Addicts are encased in a system of acquisition of a drug and the consistent reward pattern of ingestion and of decreasing awareness of other rewarding stimuli or the need to invest energies in other rewarding activities. More often, the addict maintains a limited consciousness of the destructive and alienating cycles of their addiction and only enters treatment as a result of some consequence of their use (e.g., a spouse's threat to leave, job intervention, licensing problems, legal difficulties) and rarely as a result of insight into their behavior and addiction (Ryan and Deci 2001).

Many addicts, prior to exposure to addicting agents, can be seen as running "two quarts low in feel-good chemistry." An exaggerated reward response occurs when the predisposed addict finds their drug (or behavior) or drugs of choice. These feel-good chemicals are produced rapidly and in overabundance. A unique exaggerated reward response, or "high," is the outcome of this deficit and sensitivity to mood-altering agents. This overabundance is only temporary. In fact, the addict's brain soon adapts to the rewards and eventually produces less feel-good chemical than before the whole cycle started. The brain basically fatigues in the face of this onslaught of good feeling. So the addict simply stops using at this point, right? Wrong. Once this addiction train is out of the station, stopping it is no small feat. The part of the brain that can put the brakes on (the prefrontal cortex) is increasingly cut out of the process.

Baker and Greenberg (2007) stated that from an evolutionary standpoint, humans actually have three brains. The first is the most primitive is referred to as the reptilian brain, and consists of the brain stem and lower brain, areas focused on survival. It is similar to what is seen in reptiles, like snakes. The second is the mammalian or limbic brain, which came about with the evolution of mammals. It is the brain responsible for the desire to run in packs, as survival was easier when collective strength was involved. Emotions like love, anger, compassion, jealousy, and hope and the complexities that arose from becoming socially connected are possible because of evolution of the limbic/mammalian brain.

Finally, humans developed a higher-order-thinking brain that involved social aspects of law, morality, and civility. This third brain is referred to as the neocortex (especially the frontal areas), which allows modern humans to put the brakes on what the other two brains may do much more automatically. It is responsible for our ability to reflect, have self-awareness, and make decisions.

While in addiction, the brain is dictated by more primitive instinct-driven processes as opposed to higher-order functioning in the prefrontal cortex (neocortex) regarding choice. The sidelining of this decision-making part of the brain can actually be observed in sophisticated imaging techniques like fMRI and PET scanning. This is the neurological expression of hedonic adaptation. The addict is constitutionally prone to hedonic adaptation and the hedonic treadmill and needs to work harder than others to reverse this tendency. In order to effectively accomplish this, the addict must know, with some precision, their personality functions, strengths, and weaknesses. Chapter 5, "Who Are You? Personality and Addiction," will assist in this discovery, and with "What Are You Looking For?" (Chapter 6) and "What Makes You Happy?" (Chapter 7), a pattern is created that is unique for every individual. This pattern interacts with triggers and recovery strategies that together create a fluid system that naturally shifts with the moment-to-moment fluctuations of daily life. A healthy balance within the dynamics of this system allows for the possibility of continued growth and a positive sobriety.

# 2. Understanding the Disease of Addiction

*Addiction is a Brain Disease*
(Alan Leshner PhD, Director, NIDA, 1996)

The concept of alcoholism and other drug dependency as being a disease first surfaced early in the nineteenth century. In 1956, the American Medical Association (AMA) declared alcoholism an illness. However, it wasn't until 1987 that the AMA and other medical organizations officially termed addiction a disease. Today, the concept of addiction as a disease has widespread acceptance. The American Society of Addiction Medicine (ASAM) created a public policy statement (2011) that captures the essence of our current understanding:

> *Addiction is a primary, chronic disease of brain reward, motivation, memory and related circuitry. Dysfunction in these circuits leads to characteristic biological, psychological, social and spiritual manifestations. This is reflected in an individual pathologically pursuing reward and/or relief by substance use and other behaviors.*
>
> *Addiction is characterized by inability to consistently abstain, impairment in behavioral control, craving, diminished recognition of significant problems with one's behaviors and interpersonal relationships, and a dysfunctional emotional response. Like other chronic diseases, addiction often involves cycles of relapse and remission. Without treatment or engagement in recovery activities, addiction is progressive and can result in disability or premature death.*

This description of the disease of addiction has definite utility when trying to understand the mechanisms responsible for the processes that occur under the direct influence of substances or addicting behaviors and for a period of time in early abstinence. The phenomenon of craving in some people can also be at least partly attributed to these neurophysiologic mechanisms. Under the direct influence of the disease, the addict is in an altered state of consciousness, one that is now measurable newer imaging techniques. When an addict is not using but close in time to use or triggered to use, there is a pull toward this altered state. This is like a gravitational pull that is particularly strong in the addict. It can help to know this, as it helps explain what can uniquely happen in the addict. This can help with denial as well as shame that often accompany use and craving states and most certainly relapse. There are also advantages for the medical community to understand these mechanisms so that the proper specialized approaches to addiction can be implemented. The status of "disease" can also assist with the necessary coverage for treatment, giving addiction the rightful parity with other diseases in psychiatry and medicine. But a strong word of caution is necessary.

The disease model can limit the growth in character and self-awareness that need to occur in a positive sobriety. In fact, the emphasis of this book is to recognize our inherent capacity to rise above and positively influence our physiology. So, as important as the following understanding of the disease is, the limitations of the disease model that end this section need to be fully understood.

Addiction can be defined as the continued use of a mood-altering, addicting substance or behavior (e.g., gambling, compulsive sexual behaviors) despite adverse consequences. Professionals have learned that alcoholism is a primary, chronic disease with genetic, psychosocial, and environmental factors influencing its development and manifestations. It is characterized by continuous or periodic impaired control over addicting substances despite adverse consequences, and distortions in thinking, most notably denial. This is a definition forwarded in the *Journal of the American Medical Association* in 1992, and it includes the thinking of the American Society of Addiction Medicine and the National Council on Alcoholism and Drug Dependencies. Since 1992, continued exploration of the nature of addiction has included other mood-altering substances besides alcohol as well as a number of highly reinforcing behaviors. Additionally, the disease model implies that addicts are incapable of returning to controlled use; therefore, treatment should be focused on abstinence. The disease model of addiction is now well understood and accepted by both research and clinical professionals (Guze et al. 1986). To fully understand this disease allows one to fully appreciate the powerlessness and unmanageability that accompany it.

A percentage of the population (thought to be around 50 percent of all addicts) has a biogenetic predisposition to chemicals or addictive behaviors or both; however, early life traumatic experience such as isolation or abuse can also contribute to a predisposition to addiction. Furthermore, exposure to addicting substances for any reason can produce vulnerability to addiction. In fact, recent studies suggest that even a single exposure to a substance like morphine can make lasting changes in the brain, affecting memory and creating a process of pathological learning; that is, learning to crave drugs. Once there is excessive drug use, there are disturbances in stress response systems. This often leads to compulsive repetitive patterns in an effort to capture the initial reinforcement or to block withdrawal (Koob and Kreek 2007). The disease of addiction represents a spectrum of affected individuals. In any case, the end result is the same: repeated behaviors in the face of negative consequences.

## Genetics

Familial transmission of alcoholism risk is, in part, genetically induced (Bohman et al. 1987; Devor and Cloninger 1989; Cloninger 1987; Edenberg 2003). Animal studies have demonstrated that specific alcoholism-related traits like sensitivity to intoxication and sedative effects, development of tolerance and withdrawal, and even susceptibility to organ damage can have genetic origins. Family illness studies, twin studies, and adoption studies have all supported a genetic contribution to alcoholism. The Human Genome Project is also contributing to our understanding of the role of genetics in alcoholism. The National Institute on Alcohol Abuse and Alcoholism's (NIAAA) Collaborative Study on the Genetics of Alcoholism discovered reduced brain wave amplitude in subjects that reflects an underlying genetic variation in the brain's response to alcohol (National Institute on Alcohol Abuse and Alcoholism 2003). Genetic variants referred to as "polymorphisms" are being intensively studied. Some of these variants, like those that determine the metabolism of alcohol dehydrogenase, can protect some people from alcoholism by producing a flushing response (like a natural antabuse reaction). Other polymorphisms involved in this same pathway, like ADH2 and 3, seem to predispose those who possess them to alcoholism.

What has been demonstrated in alcoholism has generally held true for other abused substances and addicting behaviors. For example, beta-endorphin levels may be low in predisposed individuals with an exaggerated response to alcohol (van den Wildenberg, Wiers, and Dessers 2007) and opiates. The stronger urge to drink in the alcoholic may be related to the G allele that predisposes the individual to drug use in general (Gianoulakis, Krishnan, and Thavundayil 1996). There are certain polymorphisms or genetic variations such as with the A1 allele of the D2 receptor gene (OPRMI) that may result in reduced dopamine signaling leading to greater need for artificial means for dopamine enhancement (Parsian, Cloninger, and Zhang 2000). These genetic variations may also predict responses to certain medications. For example, naltrexone may work much better in this A1 variation group, even possibly stimulating "hidden opiate receptors," thereby producing a paradoxical sense of well-being (Kosten et al. 2002). Sometimes, for some alcoholics, a paradoxical response that occurs has been referred to as "endorphin sensitive alcoholism" and may be seen in up to one-third of alcoholics with a northern European background (Heilig et al. 2011). This group tends to have a good response to naltrexone.

Other genetic variations that involve, for example, the GABA, neuropeptide Y, and glutamate systems are implicated in multiple addiction scenarios. Some of these are linked with personality variable, age of likely onset of addiction, and vulnerability to stress and depression. The future of addiction medicine will be closely linked to these specific variants, providing an even greater ability for individualized treatments. It also appears that drug of choice is at least in part determined in many by genetic variants (see the chart on the following page).

**Positive Sobriety**

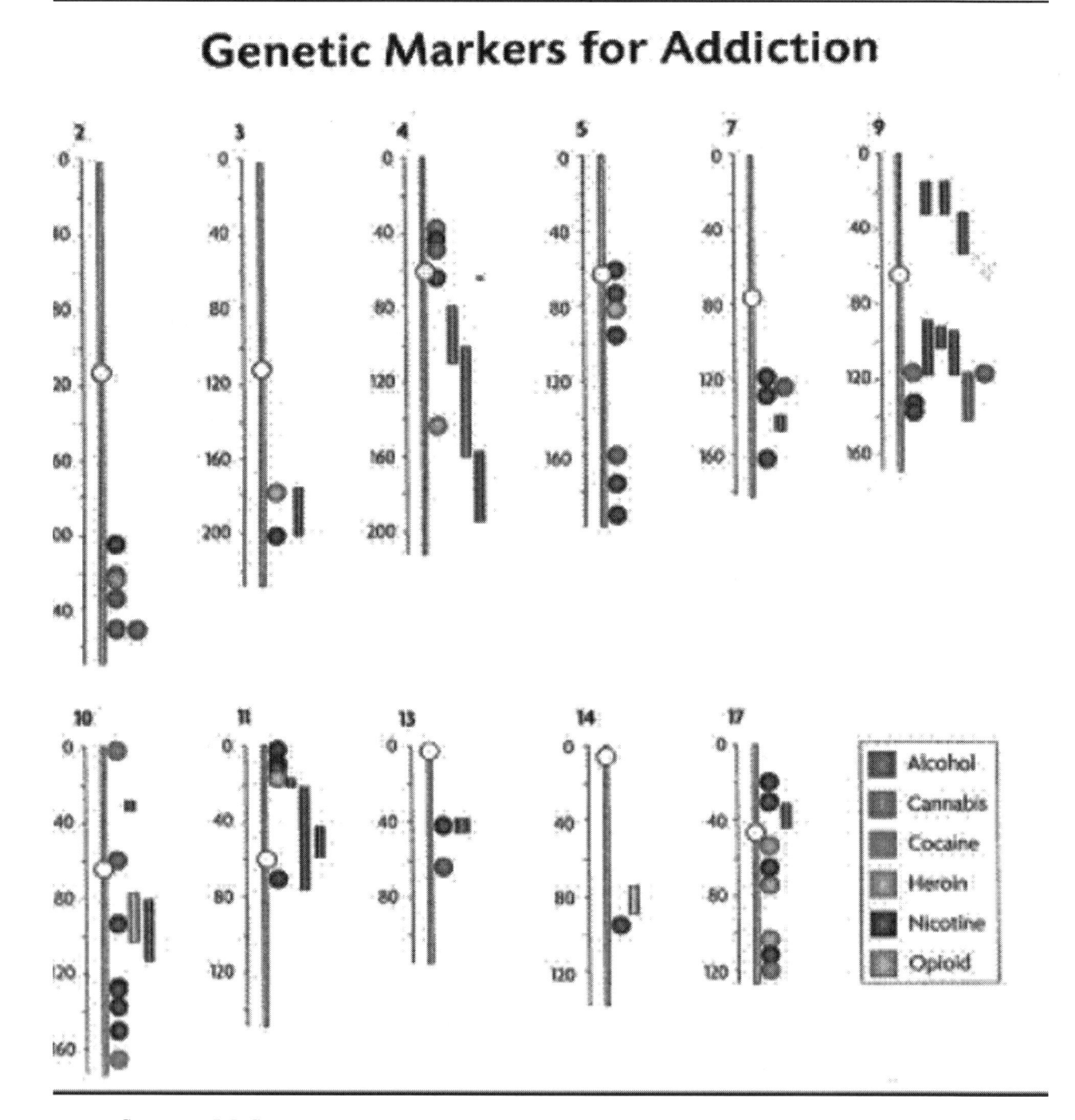

# Genetic Markers for Addiction

Sweeney, M. S. 2009. *Brain: The complete mind*. Washington, D.C.: National Geographic.

## 2. Understanding the Disease of Addiction

In a 2003 editorial in *The American Journal of Psychiatry* titled "Predisposition to Addiction: Pharmacokinetics, Pharmacodynamics and Brain Circuitry," Dr. Peter Kalivas states, "There is little doubt that the development of addiction to drugs of abuse is in part a function of predisposing factors in an individual's genome as well as factors associated with childhood and adolescent development." Furthermore, more research is pointing to the commonality of all addictive processes, whether substance or behavioral in origin. This concept will be discussed in more detail later on. It is important to note that genetic vulnerability doesn't ensure addiction. These vulnerabilities still need to be expressed (gene expression), and that depends on many factors, including environment, personality, and comorbid illnesses like depression.

In the article, "Personality Traits and Vulnerability or Resilience to Substance Use Disorders" (Belcher and Volkow et.al 2014) the authors describe that genes that moderate personality traits and how they interact with the environment and drugs may give us the best clues as to susceptibility in becoming an addict.

It is the disease model that informs treatment programs that address the psychosocial and environmental factors that contributed to the addictive behaviour in an attempt to combat the genetic influences. In fact, current evidence has suggested that 50 to 60 percent of addiction is genetically informed, leaving 40 to 50 percent to environmental and psychosocial factors (Dick and Bierut 2006).

The combination of the treatment interventions described throughout this manual addresses that remaining 40 to 50 percent. The goal of treatment is to replace the addiction with personal growth and satisfaction with lifestyle, or a *positive sobriety*.

### Plainly Stated

**Those studying addiction have taken great strides in understanding addiction as a biogenetic disease. The genetics of this disease is highly complex, and there will be continued study for some time to come. One finding does stand out: genetics plays a role in most that are addicted. It appears to explain the unique reaction—that "magical connection"—most addicts feel when they use initially. It may explain drug (and behavior) of choice and even associated psychological issues like depression, anxiety, or even some personality dysfunctions as genetic subtypes. This is giving us an important way of understanding the unique presentations of this disease and allowing for more targeted treatments. Environment and experience (like prolonged stress) also shape the brain along with the use of drugs themselves. We always need to remember that genes are important but are not the only reason addiction occurs. When involved, genes are expressed in an environment that promotes that expression.**

# Reward

The reward circuitry of the brain involves the mesolimbic dopamine system including the prefrontal cortex, the nucleus accumbens, and the ventral tegmental (VTA) areas of the brain.

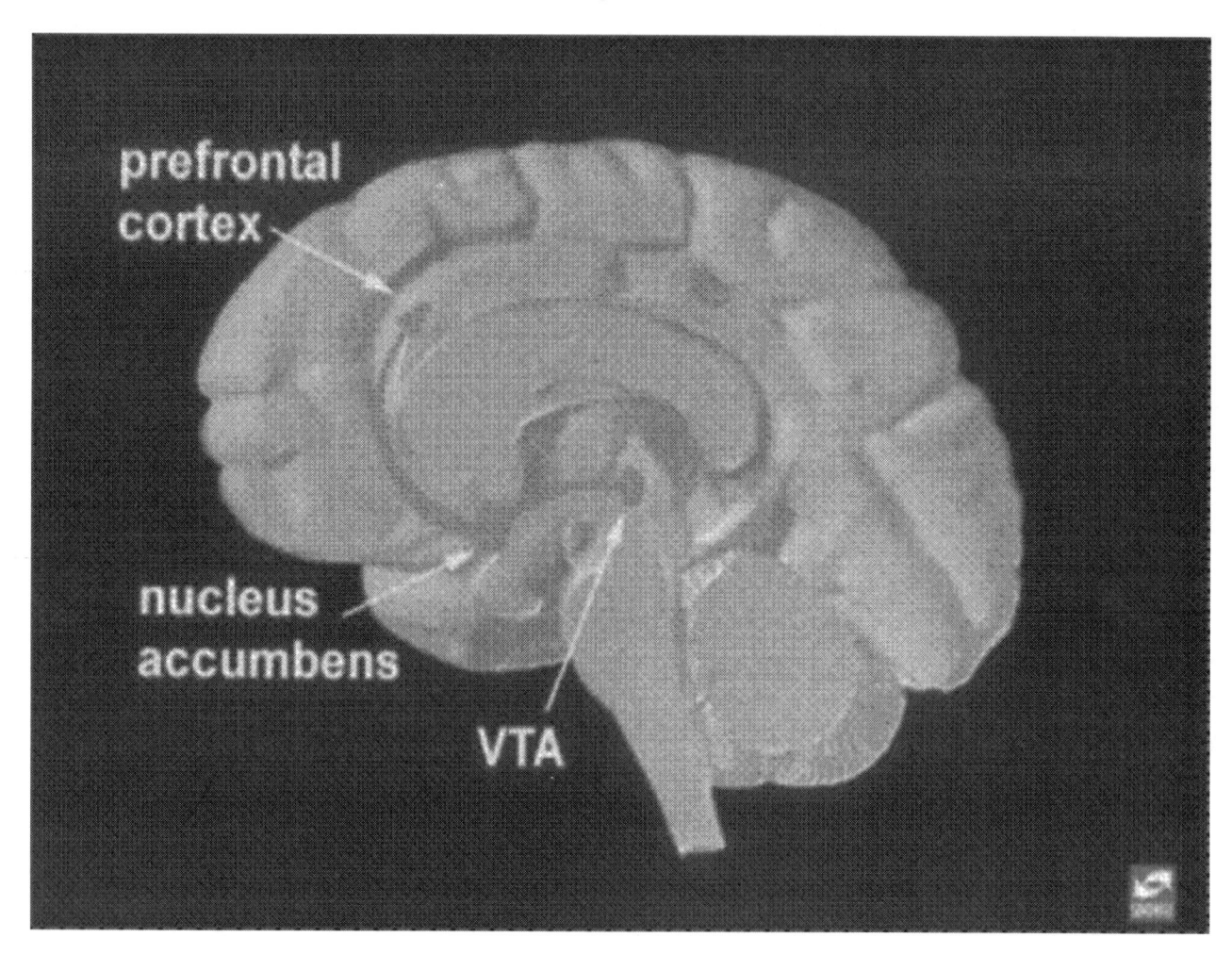

The mesolimbic pathways connect the more automatic bodily functions of the brain stem and peripheral nervous system and the emotional, or limbic, areas of the brain to the prefrontal cortex, which is the thinking or reflective and decision-making part of the central nervous system. Happiness doesn't come in a bottle, pill, powder, or morsel. Intellectually, everyone knows that. The brain reward circuitry people possess does not catch on to this fact as quickly. In fact, what underlies addiction is this reward problem. "Reward" is the term neuroscience uses to describe experiences that bear repeating, like pleasure or relief from some discomfort. Neuroscience has come a long way in specifically identifying the areas of the brain involved in reward (the brain reward circuitry) and the neurochemistry (our "feel-good chemicals") that create these reward responses (e.g., dopamine and beta-endorphins). Neurotransmitters (including dopamine and beta-endorphins) facilitate the communication of these systems in the reward center. This pathway is involved in essential behaviors such as eating, sleeping, and sex and is essentially hijacked in the addict. This pleasure pathway in the brain, which we share with other animals, was discovered by Dr. James Olds who, through electrical stimulation of this pleasure center (specifically the hypothalamus), demonstrated that lab animals will self-stimulate this area and completely ignore food and water in the process (1956).

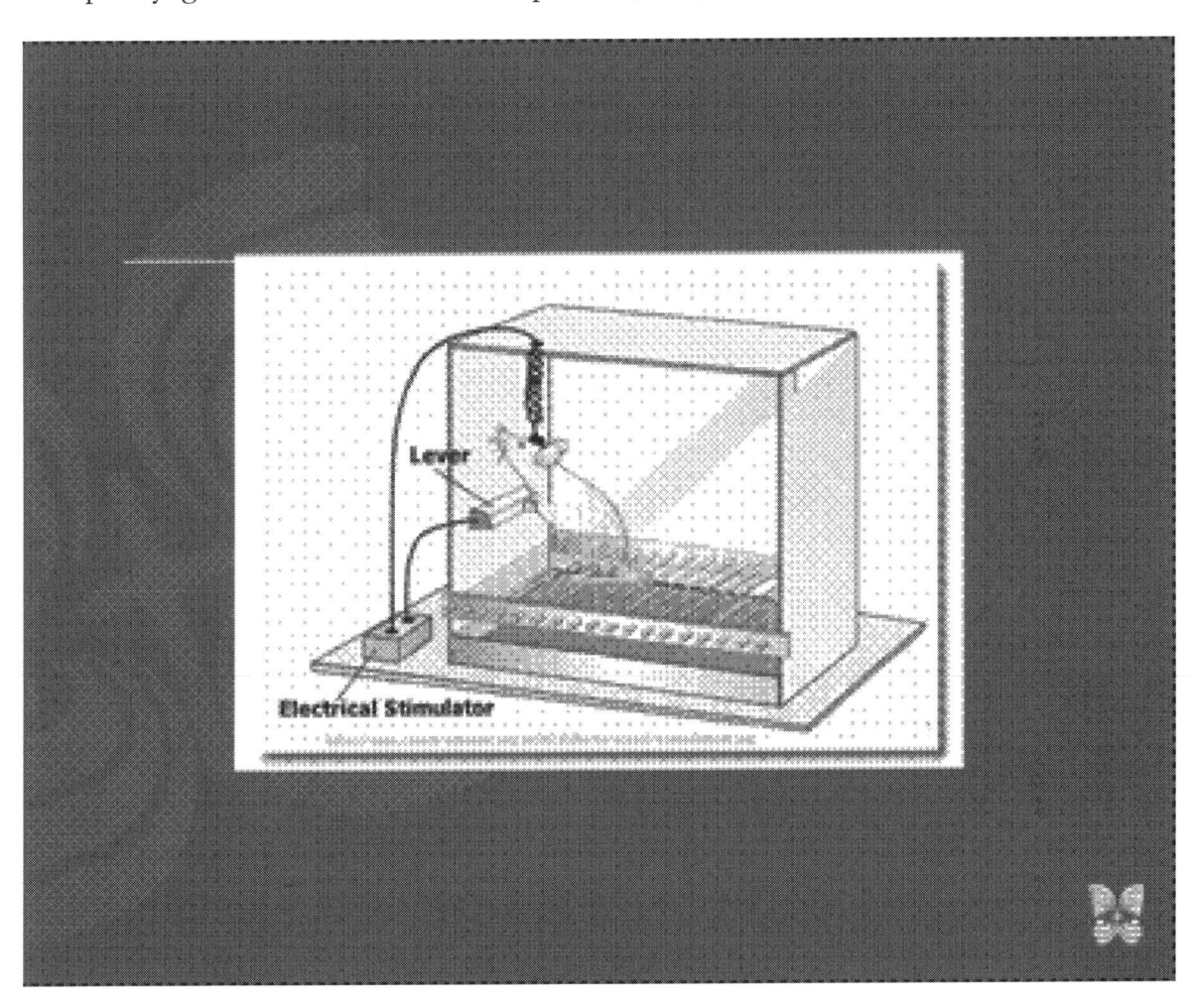

The addict's initial motivation is to feel pleasure. Eventually the reward pathway shifts its sensitivities to the substance or behavior instead of the internal neurotransmitters.

The initial experience of drug use for some people can be described as a "magical connection." The predisposed brain of the addict can be like a lock with the addicting substances (or behaviors) of choice representing the key. This vulnerability, as previously discussed, may have a genetic component or be shaped by environment or both. In any case, the drug does something to the person that "hooks" them. In some cases where this initial connection may not occur but where repeated use happens anyway (for example, through peer pressure), the brain responds to the repeated use by shifts in the reward system that over time create this unique connection. In either case, the experience that opens the door is extremely and abnormally powerful, even "magical," in its effects.

Many addicts describe this initial experience as finally feeling "normal." Sometimes a paradoxical (opposite) response occurs, such as an opiate like hydrocodone or alcohol (both sedating drugs) producing stimulation and increased energy. This is one reason so many health care professionals addicted to oral painkillers describe initially feeling these drugs help them be more alert. Consequently, they feel they can work more hours and even be more effective at what they do, which in turn feeds their denial that their use is a problem. This initial connection is relatively short-lived. Invariably, a vicious cycle is produced. In the pursuit of reward, the receptors that naturally mediate reward become desensitized or diminished, creating the need for more substances, contributing to tolerance and withdrawal. The more the addict uses, the more they need, creating the progressive, vicious cycle that is the hallmark of all addictions (Berridge and Kringelbach 2008).

**Plainly Stated**

**The brain reward center is now well understood. It plays a critical role in the relationship between addict and substance (or behavior). On one hand this reward center is essential for the experience of pleasure and our survival as a species. Unfortunately, it is hijacked in addiction, which explains why the addict continues in the addiction despite adverse consequences.**

# Learning and Memory

Learning and memory faculties are negatively impacted in addictive behaviors. Hyman (2005) defines addiction in terms of learning and memory and discusses the impact of addictive behaviors in usurping the neural mechanisms of learning and memory that under normal circumstances shape survival behaviors related to pursuit of rewards and predictive cues. If survival is too intimately associated in the addict's mind with securing the substance of use, then rewards and predictive cues are developed around the substance. Chronic substance use results in impaired reward-related learning, to the extent that addicts may believe that the hedonic properties of the substance far exceed any other goals and thereby devote their lives to attaining the substance.

Dopamine, a powerful neurotransmitter, can shape stimulus-reward learning, or the behavioral response to reward-related stimuli. Cueing involves significant associational memories, and connectionist brain theory suggests that these associations are wired into the brain. For example, a patient placed in the environment in which they previously used a substance may be vulnerable to an emerging pattern of brain stimuli and connections that can motivate the patient to use.

Long-term potentiation, or LTP, is an important concept in learning. Like long-term memory, LTP involves the strengthening of the connections between neurons secondary to repeated exposures. Researchers are studying LTP and recognizing that addiction represents a powerful form of learning and memory. As previously stated, addiction is a complex neurobehavioral disease involving various parts of the brain reward circuitry, such as the ventral tegmental area (VTA) and nucleus accumbens (NAc). Studies have demonstrated that VTA and NAc synapses are capable of undergoing LTP (Kauer and Malenka 2007) and that this LTP may be responsible for the behaviors that characterize addiction (Wolf 2003).

Because of the power of addiction in this reward center, this research suggests a circular pattern of reinforcement with diminished capacity for the addict to incorporate new learning strategies. Addicts are encased in a system of acquisition of a drug and the consistent reward pattern of ingestion, with decreasing awareness of other rewarding stimuli or the need to invest energy in other rewarding activities. More often, the addict maintains a limited consciousness of the destructive and alienating cycles of addiction and only comes into treatment as a result of some consequence of use (e.g., spouse's threat to leave, job intervention, licensing problems, legal difficulties, and so on) and rarely as a result of insight into their behavior and addiction.

The individual with an addictive disease who has engaged in chronic substance use will maintain a series of intact or collaboratively fragmented memories of the addictive behaviors and will likely recall these memories with ease during periods of craving. Memories of successful sobriety and newly learned behaviors have not likely been practiced with the same level of intensity in early recovery and are therefore vulnerable to being overridden. Also, addicts will experience a period of time referred to as "post-acute withdrawal" early in sobriety. The most common symptoms are lack of concentration, irritability, and insomnia. (See "Core Treatment Lectures and Workshops" for more information about post-acute withdrawal).

The addict has adopted a reactive response to feeling uncomfortable, and that reaction is to use a substance. Addicts will need physiological, psychological, and social support to counteract their impulsive need to medicate these uncomfortable states. Educational support is also critical, but education alone will not deter an addict from relapse. Physiological changes that impact behavior do not respond to the intellect, and the very engagement in extended addictive behaviors minimize the power of the individual's will, which results in cyclical and self-rewarding patterns of addiction.

## Motivation

Motivation is another factor with biological components, and the pursuit of goals that produce desired outcomes is an integral aspect of addiction and recovery. Kalivas and Volkow (2005) support the theory that addiction involves a dysregulation in the motive circuitry, and the repetitive use of addictive drugs reorganizes brain circuitry to establish behaviors characteristic of addiction. PET studies on cue-induced craving clearly demonstrate increased reactions between the amygdala and the prefrontal cortex when people are actively reminded of their addicting agent. The next graphic shows how cues such as pictures of drug paraphernalia activate the prefrontal cortex's dorsolateral (DL) area and the amygdala (AM). The prefrontal cortex, responsible for decision making, gets activated with the amygdala, the fear-based part of the brain, creating a connection for craving. This activates a neurotransmitter called glutamate, which creates an unpleasant feeling associated with craving that can cause the addict to try and reduce this discomfort through drug use.

## Positive Sobriety

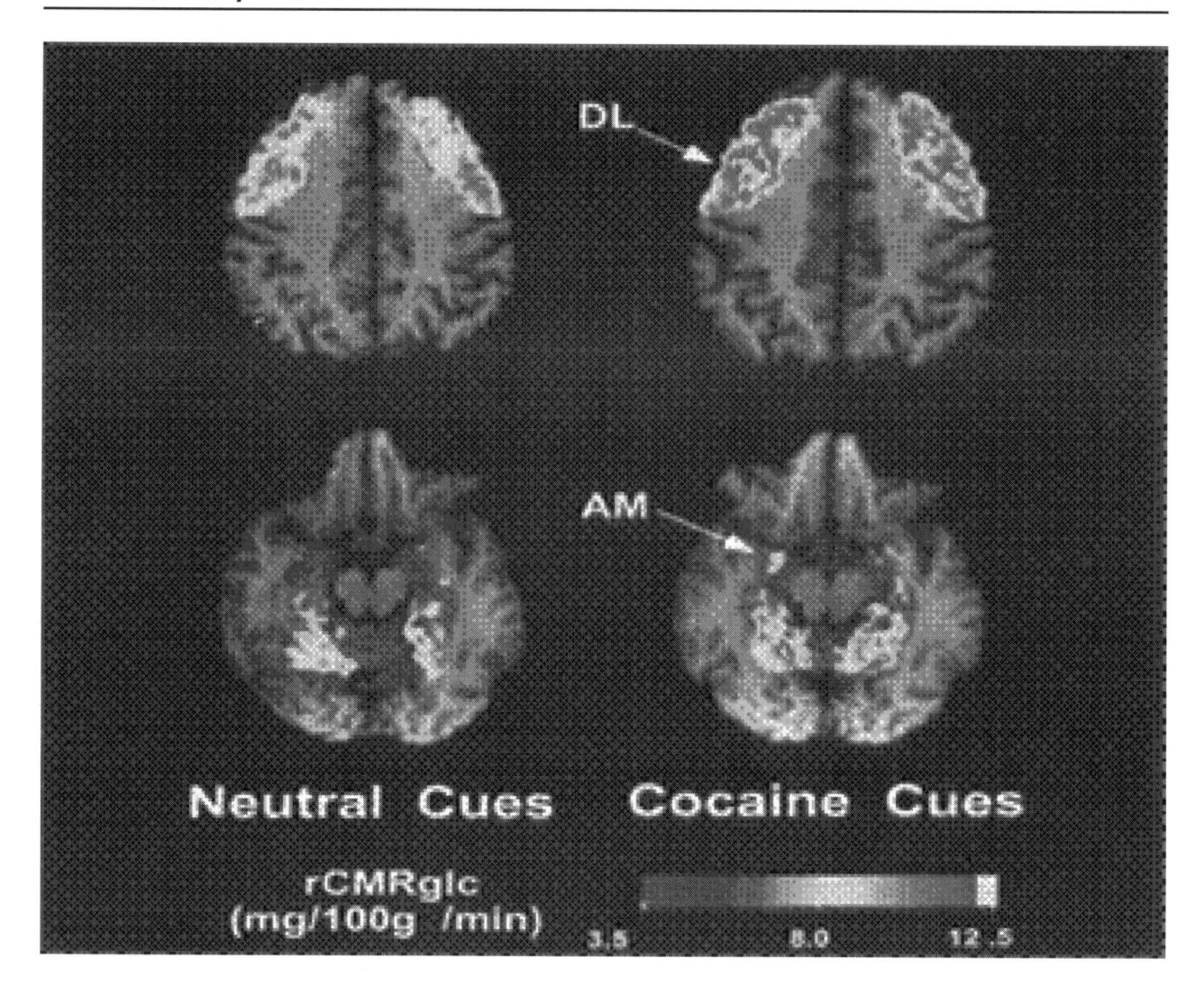

From Kaufman 2001

In addition to the obvious consequences of engaging in addictive behavior (i.e., legal, financial, psychosocial), there is a risk of neuronal recircuiting that results in physiological cycles of addictive behaviors, and these circuits are increasingly difficult to break. Kalivas and Volkow (2005) propose three temporally distinct phases of addiction:

Stage 1: Acute Drug Effects

Stage 2: Transition to Addiction

Stage 3: End-Stage Addiction

In stage 1, acute drug administration results in molecular consequences that are widely distributed in the brain circuitry that impact motivation. Stage 2 reflects neuronal changes, such as D1-receptor-mediated stimulation of proteins. Stage 3 introduces the possibility that changes in protein content, function, or both move from temporary to permanent features. The researchers concluded that cellular adaptations in the prefrontal glutamatergic innervation of the accumbens are responsible for the promotion of compulsive-character drug seeking in addicts through decreasing the value of natural rewards, reducing cognitive control (choice), and increasing glutamatergic drive in response to drugs and association with drugs. In other words, the addict's brain progresses to a point where it is driven to use, sensing that only use will bring pleasure, while having diminished ability to find healthy ways to receive reward (e.g., connection with people or spiritual pursuits).

# Decision Making

Decision making is another area of cognitive function negatively impacted by addictive behaviors. A publication in *Psychiatry* (Noel, van der Linden, and Bechara 2006) suggested that addiction is an imbalance between the neural system that is reactive for signaling pain or pleasure and another neural system that is reflective and controls the reactive system. When the ventromedial prefrontal cortex (VMPC) is injured in patients who are not addicts, they make disadvantageous decisions and fail to learn from their mistakes, contrary to their preinjury personalities. The authors made striking comparisons between patients with VMPC injuries and addicts: both deny they have a problem and appear to ignore the consequences of their actions. In addiction, the neural mechanisms that enable an individual to reflect and choose wisely appear to be weakened, and they move from self-directed behavior to automatic sensory-driven behavior. The authors hypothesized that for certain people, the decision-making mechanism—the process by which one reflects and considers consequences prior to an action—in the brain is weak, and this weakness makes them vulnerable to addiction. The source of the weakness can be genetic or environmentally induced, but it is always a consequence of addiction. *Two decision-making areas of the brain are particularly affected in addiction: the orbitofrontal cortex, involved in deciding what is really best for us, and the anterior cingulate cortex, which helps us understand if the decision we made was the right one. Both these pathways are disrupted in addiction, which invariably leads to making bad decisions and, to some degree, not even realizing the decision was bad.*

Recent fMRI and PET studies demonstrate a split between the ability to make appropriate decisions as the compulsive drive for the chemical or addiction progresses. Goldstein and Volkow (2002) demonstrated that as addiction progresses, one's ability to make appropriate choices diminishes. Increased impulsivity is accompanied by old memories of times when the addiction "worked" as well as by negation of options other than engaging in the addiction. Not only are some addicts predisposed to a sluggish reward circuitry before ever using a substance or engaging in addiction, but they also now appear to have some degree of difficulty in decision making. Deficits in the aforementioned areas constitute the vicious cycle of addiction

## Positive Sobriety

### The Vicious Cycle of Addiction

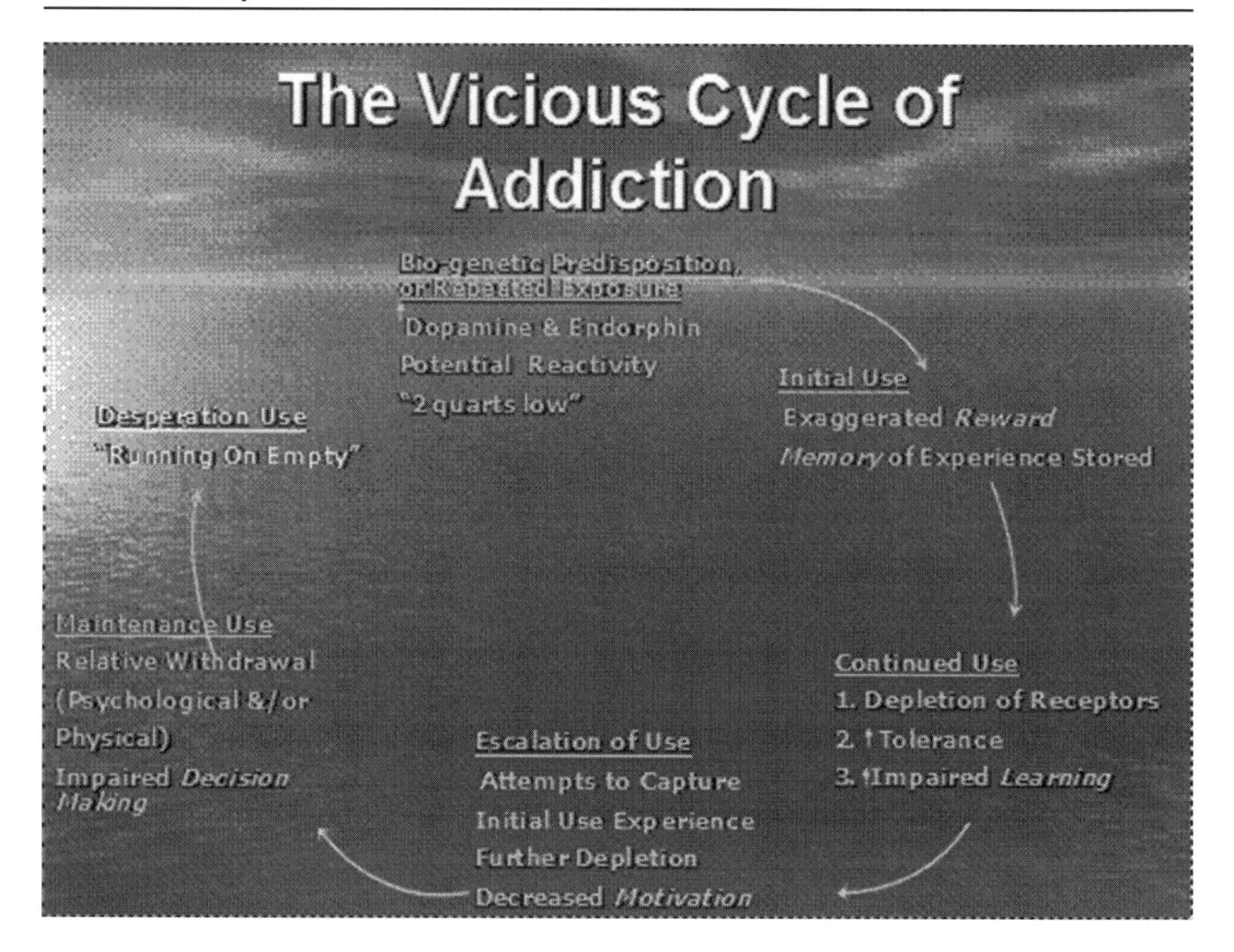

**Bio-genetic Predisposition, or Repeated Exposure:**
Dopamine & Endorphin Potential Reactivity
"2 quarts low"

**Initial Use**
Exaggerated *Reward*
*Memory* of Experience Stored

**Continued Use**
1. Depletion of Receptors
2. ↑Tolerance
3. ↑Impaired *Learning*

**Escalation of Use**
Attempts to Capture Initial Use Experience
Further Depletion
Decreased *Motivation*

**Maintenance Use**
Relative Withdrawal (Psychological &/or Physical)
Impaired *Decision Making*

**Desperation Use**
"Running On Empty"

Figure 1: The above figure outlines how a predisposition (being "two quarts low") creates a vicious cycle through initial intensified reward and continued and escalating use. The more one uses, the more they need, and the more they need, the more they use and the more they shut down their own endogenous feel-good chemistry, leading to a downward spiral. Increasing deficits in learning, memory, motivation, and decision making accompany this process, accelerating the downward spiral.

Plainly Stated

Addiction may start with that magical connection, often referred to as "Reward Sensitivity" but other factors quickly take over. These include issues with memory, learning, motivation, and decision making. Over time, repeated use stores the memory deep in various parts of the brain, especially the ones associated with strong emotion. It is as if we learn to be addicted and learn it too well! The motivation for use becomes overwhelming, and eventually, as the disease progresses, we lose our ability to make decisions—in a sense, our disease makes them for us. This is particularly related to triggers or 'cues' and referred to as "Cue Sensitivity" The disease and its progression can be summarized as "Reward Sensitivity and Cue Reactivity". Recovery involves a whole new learning process: one that needs to be strong enough to overcome the power of addiction.

## Behavioral Addictions and Addictive Interactive Disorders

Today, we have a much more global understanding of the disease of addiction. Through modern research methods, including neuroimaging, we see that some compulsive behaviors such as overeating, gambling, and sexual behaviors can also represent addictions. For example, in June 2011, *Discover* magazine reported the work of Dr. Eric Stice at the Oregon Research Center. He performed fMRI scans on compulsive overeaters and found that a DNA polymorphism (like we discussed previously with genetics and chemical addiction) related to reduced signaling dopamine (less capacity for reward) was more prevalent in this group, causing them to eat more to get pleasure. This has been confirmed in animal studies as well (Johnson and Kinney 2010).

These behavioral addictions seem to interact on the same reward pathways as do addicting substances, producing the same addicting patterns. Genetics can play a role as well. For example, as we can see in chemical addiction, a DNA polymorphism can cause a lack of reward responsiveness in the dopamine receptor gene that in turn can facilitate compulsive overeating.

There are other addictive patterns that are sometimes referred to as "soft addictions." These include compulsive shopping, exercise, or Internet games such as World of Warcraft. They can be disabling, and further research is being done to see what effect they have on the reward circuitry.

As early as the nineteenth century, there are references in medical texts to the interaction between addictions. It was called "intemperance," and stated that the use of alcohol and tobacco would lead to excessive eating, sexual behavior, and other misadventures. A more recent term, Addiction interactive disorder (AID) (Carnes 2004) implies that addiction has many forms, such as gambling, food, sex, work, certain financial behaviors, and even religiosity. Addictions do not just coexist; they reinforce, intensify, or become part of the rituals of the chemical addiction. Of course, they may create their own powerful addiction independent of chemical addiction as well.

A major factor in relapse in chemical dependency is the failure to recognize and treat companion addictions that are a part of the addictive process. AID is fairly common in addicted populations. Bill W., cofounder of Alcoholics Anonymous, suffered from compulsive sexual behavior and financial disorders after he became sober from alcohol (1976).

A percentage of patients with chemical dependency also meets criteria for other compulsive behaviors or addictions. For this reason, all patients in primary care treatment need to be screened for other addictions. The definition may be simple: that the individual engages in the addictive behavior despite adverse consequences. However, the patient must meet strict criteria in a formal screening before a diagnosis is made. Also, input from others, such as a spouse or other close family members, are helpful since many patients are protective and secretive about these behaviors and are ambivalent or skeptical about AID and its need to be treated.

Blum and colleagues (1996) described a reward deficiency syndrome that includes not only alcoholism and drug addiction but also other compulsive behaviours such as gambling, sexual compulsivity, and compulsive overeating. They hypothesized that a variant (A1 allele) of the dopamine D2 receptor mediates many compulsive behaviours. Often these behavioural addictions are covert and responsible for relapse, but they can also initially lead to the chemical addiction. Carnes (2004) reinforced this more global view of addiction with an emphasis on sexual compulsivity as a devastating, progressive process that can coexist with, or be independent of, substance abuse or dependence. Huebner (1993) also informed the AID perspective by arguing that the neuroscience includes deprivation. Huebner's concept of compulsive avoidance shares the same dopamine reward system, but it is more than mere avoidance. Addicts become preoccupied and obsessed with the behaviors and ignore the life-threatening consequences, much like people with anorexia nervosa or compulsive athleticism do. These are people in patterns of extreme living. Huebner further proposed that addictions interact at primary levels and thus share etiology and structure. As such, addiction must be treated as a full spectrum disorder, not in a piecemeal approach.

One of the dimensions of AID is *replacement*. This is the process in which one addiction replaces another as the *primary* addiction. Since the neuroscience is the same, it is imperative that addicts are educated to understand the potential of replacing chemical dependency with another addiction. Other addictions often emerge six to twelve months after sobriety from mood-altering substances. Another dimension is *ritualizing*, which refers to rituals performed in association with the substance use or behavior, such as coming home from work and grabbing a beer out of the fridge before you sit down in front of the television. When rituals for one addiction are the same as or overlap with another, there is an interaction between addictions. Some people combine drinking alcohol with smoking cigarettes. All addictive behaviors have the effect of numbing or stress reduction for the addict, however short-lived and potentially deadly.

Carnes (2004) states the need for all addictions to be treated aggressively. He gives three clinical strategies:

1) The time line

2) The neuropathic interview

3) The self-assessment workshop

The time line refers to the task of the patient to create a time line of the major events in their life, including the onset of each addiction, worst moments, and other notable moments. This will give a visual and concrete representation of the addiction and interactions to the patients and treatment team. The neuropathic interview begins with educating the patient on the neuropathways of the brain so the individual might bypass the shame that keeps the behaviors secret and arrive at an intellectual understanding of AID. The counselor asks questions and collects data to present the patterns of addiction and the effect and purpose of the phases of the addiction and finally to help the addict identify their triggers for the behaviour. The last strategy, the self-assessment, is a standardized list of criteria rated by the addict from which they learn the common characteristics of addictions. The result is gaining insight about the power of addictions and learning to identify how addictions interact to make one vulnerable to relapse. Hopefully, the patient is open to recovery from all addictions, since a relapse in one addiction often causes a relapse in another. The recommendations for continued recovery closely follow the same recommendations for chemical dependency recovery, including commitment to a twelve-step program such as Gamblers Anonymous, Sexaholics Anonymous, Overeaters Anonymous, and others, and an ongoing commitment to nonchemical coping skills, such as meditation, therapy, optimal nutrition, and an exercise program.

In the positive sobriety program we have an expert in AID issues consult with us, give lectures, assess patients for AID, and run a weekly AID-focused group. This is enough for some, but others may need for a formal treatment program to address AID in a comprehensive and focused way and to help the patient detoxify from the discomfort they often feel in early recovery.

# Nicotine Dependence

Nicotine use and dependence has historically been separated from addiction to alcohol and other drugs like cocaine and opiates in treatment programs. Although nicotine does not create the high of these other substances, it is a major health issue and can negatively impact outcomes, and it needs to be aggressively addressed in treatment.

Nicotine use in treatment populations is three times higher than in the general population. People often minimize the dangerousness of nicotine because it generally results in no short-term consequences, no job impairment, no legal consequences, and no family or marital problems. Addressing use of this substance while in treatment is important, as smoking-related illnesses are the highest cause of death in people in recovery. In fact, smoking-related illnesses are responsible for about 443,000 deaths in the United States (49,400 of which are due to secondhand smoke) and 5 million deaths worldwide annually. It is the most preventable cause of death and results in an average loss of 13 to 14 years of life compared to nonsmokers. It is estimated that 25 million Americans will die prematurely from smoking-related illnesses, including 5 million younger than 18 years of age (Centers for Disease Control and Prevention 2008). Smoking also has been noted to increase relapse rates in recovering addicts (Gulliver, Kamholz, and Helstrom 2006). *Addiction treatment is focused on helping addicts rediscover life and promoting healthful living*, and continuing to smoke after spending so much time and energy on this task is counterintuitive. Breaking the cycle of nicotine use in addition to breaking your other substance use cycle is an empowering experience. Many people think that quitting smoking while in a recovery program is the worst time to quit, while in fact it is the best time, as it is in congruence with realigning your life to be independent from substance use and abuse.

Nicotine works in the following ways: First, inhalation of the drug provides direct delivery to the brain, as the high concentration of capillaries in the lungs ensures maximum absorbency. As it does not need to go through a digestive process, the drug maintains its concentration. Once it reaches the brain, nicotine stimulates the release of dopamine, important for pleasurable feelings that facilitate the reward system. Dopamine is discussed throughout this book in relation to drug use and the reward pathways associated with it. Additionally, nicotine stimulates the adrenal glands, resulting in a release of adrenaline, which in turn causes a release of glucose and an increase in blood pressure, respiration, and heart rate. Smokers often find that their weight is controlled through smoking. Incidentally, for women in particular, this side effect is frequently a reason to continue smoking, either consciously or unconsciously.

Withdrawal symptoms begin within an hour of not smoking and include irritability, anxiety, cravings, disturbed sleep, increased appetite, and deficits in attention and cognition. The calming effect smokers attribute to smoking is likely due to nicotine reducing the experience of withdrawal symptoms, as research has been unable to find any qualities of nicotine itself that would directly produce that effect. In essence, the calm felt from smoking is more psychological in nature than pharmacological.

A variety of adverse health consequences are related to smoking. These include cancers of the lungs, mouth, lip, pharynx, larynx, esophagus, stomach, pancreas, cervix, kidney, ureter, and bladder; chronic obstructive pulmonary disease; emphysema; heart disease; leukemia; pneumonia; cataracts; reduced circulation; and dampened senses of taste and smell. It is possible to overdose from nicotine, which can result in death. Symptoms of nicotine overdose include vomiting, tremors, convulsions, and respiratory paralysis. Children who ingest chewing tobacco can exhibit signs of overdose. In fact, nicotine itself is extremely toxic—one drop of pure nicotine on the skin can be fatal. In addition to the negative health effects for yourself, you are also endangering those around you through secondhand smoke. Researchers are learning more about secondhand smoke and its detrimental health effects, especially on children. It has been linked to heart disease, lung and other cancers, and sudden infant death syndrome.

The good news is that many of the adverse health effects are reversible with abstinence. After twenty minutes, blood pressure and pulse rate decrease, and circulation improves so that the temperature of the hands and feet rises. After eight hours, carbon monoxide and oxygen levels in the body return to normal. Heart attack risk decreases after twenty-four hours, and after forty-eight hours, smell and taste improve. After the first month, nicotine withdrawal symptoms subside and the focus shifts to addressing psychological triggers of use rather than managing physical symptoms. After one year, heart attack risk drops to half that of smokers, while after five years, risk of stroke equals that of nonsmokers. Ten years after quitting, cancer risk drops significantly, and after fifteen years, risk of death from heart disease is the same as a nonsmoker. The Centers for Disease Control has a wealth of information on health topics related to smoking in addition to information about quitting. Their website, www.cdc.gov, is a great resource for this information.

It is difficult to quit because withdrawal occurs so quickly. Additionally, people smoke all day, and smoking often becomes synonymous with a variety of activities or situations, such as driving, drinking coffee, meals, stressful situations, or work breaks. Quitting requires having a plan to deal with not smoking in these situations and starts with removing access to cigarettes in general. Changing your routine can help break the cycle—for example, something as simple as drinking your coffee with your smoking hand can provide a different experience and help break that cycle. Prescription stop-smoking aids are available. The most common and most effective include bupropion (Wellbutrin, Zyban) and naltrexone, which help control cravings and weight gain; Chantix, which blocks nicotine receptors; and NicVax, which causes the production of antibodies to nicotine to prevent it from getting into the brain. There are potential side effects associated with prescription drugs that should be discussed with your physician. In addition to these medications, nicotine replacements such as the patch, gum, and inhaler help decrease withdrawal symptoms. Building a support network of friends, family, coworkers, and other ex-smokers is important to your success. If you try to quit but are constantly surrounded by people who smoke and encourage you to join them, it will be much harder for you to stick to your plan. Remember that it frequently takes people many tries to eventually kick the habit, but doing so ultimately gives you a longer and healthier life. The personal sense of self-efficacy (that is, confidence in your ability to succeed in quitting smoking) is what predicts success in quitting smoking. Long-term success in smoking cessation requires both your personal determination to quit and optimistic self-confidence because every drug dependence is rooted in the false and self-defeating perception that you cannot control the choices you make about how to live well.

**Plainly Stated**

**We are learning that addiction can involve more than just substances. Since the reward center of the brain processes intense reinforcing experiences like eating, sex, and gambling similar to addicting substances, it make sense that these rewarding behaviors can cause their own addictions. It now appears that, as with chemical dependency, there often is a biogenetic underpinning in many who struggle with these types if addiction. This addiction may occur in conjunction with chemical abuse or become a replacement for it once someone becomes abstinent from substances. We describe this phenomenon as AID, or addictive interactive disorder. Any of these behavioral addictions may be completely freestanding. This is sometimes referred to as a "process addiction." This now includes nicotine use and dependence. In any case, these are disabling addictions and need to be assessed and treated rigorously.**

# Hardware Problems and Hardware Solutions

*The disease model is reductionist; that is, it demonstrates how the brain influences behavior, thoughts, and feelings. This is an important part of the equation that allows us to use direct measures, like medication or even electrical stimulation, to influence brain mechanisms. These measures target the hardwiring of the brain that, in a simplistic manner, can be analogous to the hard drive of a computer. The ability for thoughts, feelings, and behavior to feedback and influence the brain can be thought of as software programming and will be discussed in the next section. Although somewhat artificial, these concepts can help us conceptualize an integrated mind, body, and spirit approach to addiction recovery.*

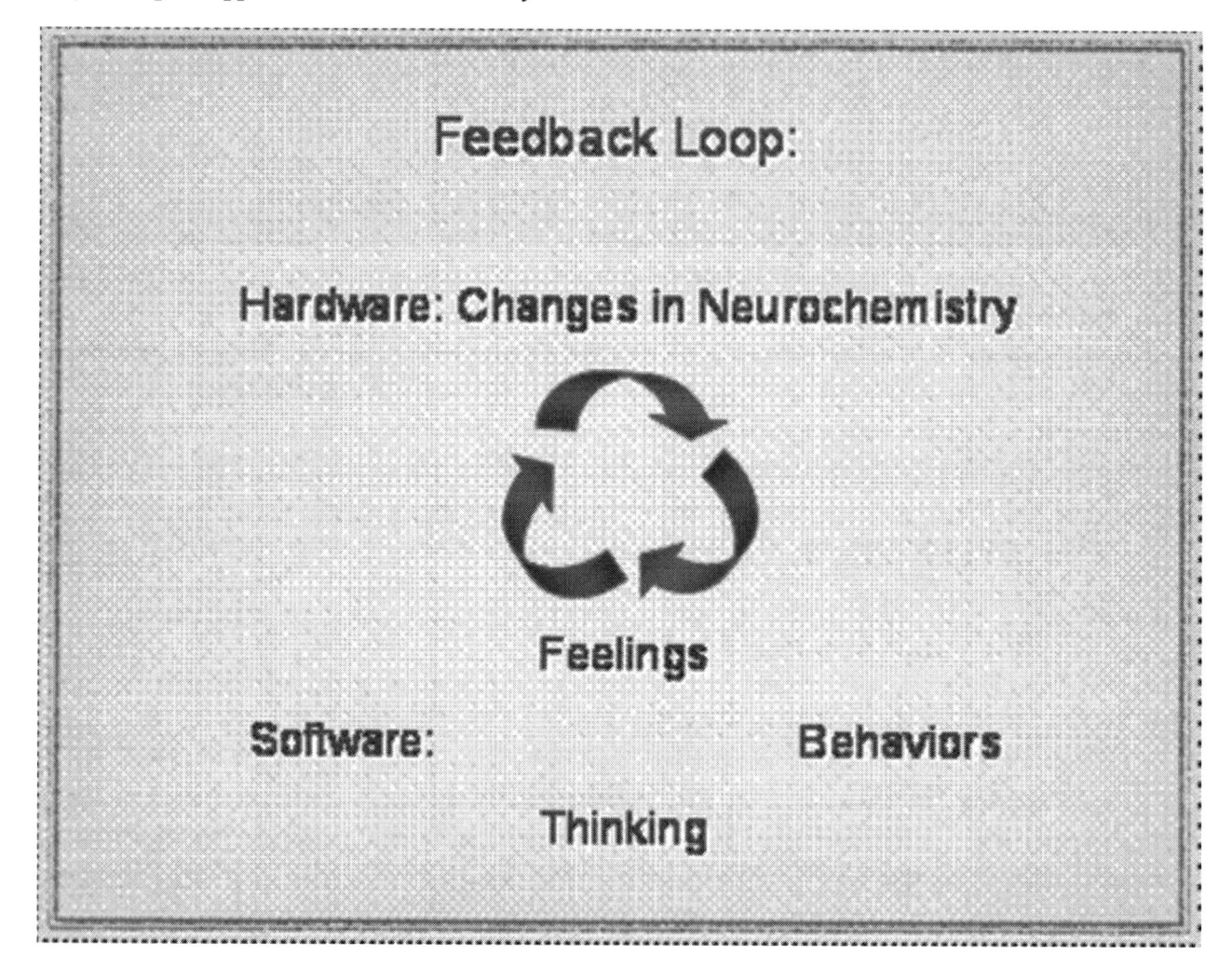

**Feedback Loop:**

**Hardware: Changes in Neurochemistry**

**Software:** Feelings Behaviors Thinking

## Hardware Treatment Interventions

Various pharmacologic interventions that target brain function can be looked at as "hardware" interventions. They involve specific medications for the addiction (e.g., to target craving or to block reward) or medication strategies for common comorbid conditions like depression or anxiety disorders. Certain conditions like ADHD, chronic pain, sleep disorders, or anxiety can be more difficult to treat since many of the medications used for these particular conditions have addicting potential.

# Specific Medications for Addiction and Comorbid Issues

## Medication Management

Medications can play a critical role in the management of addictive diseases. Anticraving medications such as acamprosate and naltrexone have proven efficacy in positive treatment outcomes. Naltrexone, which can temper craving and also block the reinforcement of alcohol and opiates, is particularly helpful for the addicted professional. For example, a health care professional addicted to opiates (e.g., an anesthesiologist) may agree to take naltrexone so they can return to a work environment in which there remains accessibility to narcotics. It enhances the confidence of the recovering addict and the workplace that agrees to reinstate or hire a newly recovering professional. An injectable form of naltrexone, Vivitrol, is now approved for alcohol and opiate dependence (there is recent discussion about efficacy in reducing stimulant intake as well) and can be administered monthly (O'Malley and Froehlich 2002; Sevarino and Kosten 2009). To date, Vivitrol has been the most useful addiction-specific medication for us. For alcoholics, naltrexone may work the best with a subgroup that are "endorphin sensitive." These are thought to be individuals of northern European extraction, and one-third of this subgroup could have a robust response to the medication, and some may even experience a mild reinforcement effect hypothesized to be from the naltrexone that facilitates hidden opiate receptors, as mentioned in the previous section on genetics. For opiate addiction, naltrexone completely occupies the opiate receptor and will block any outside opiate effect. Research suggests it will help for craving as well, and outcomes are especially good for opiate dependence (Kosten, 2002). Vivitrol is injected monthly, so compliance during that month is not an issue. It also creates a steady level in the blood, and much less of the drug has to be used. Other than injection site sensitivity in about 10 percent of patients, there are minimal side effects (such as nausea, headache, and irritability), and if present, they usually last only a day or two after the first injection. Patients may need to be on Vivitrol for a few months or several months, depending on their individual needs.

Acamprosate (Campral) is thought to modify the glutamate that can cause craving. This medication can also help with anxiety over time.

Suboxone (buprenorphine plus naloxone) is a partial agonist. It occupies the opiate receptors in the brain's reward center, partially blocking and partially activating them. This medication can produce some reinforcement initially, but that tends to diminish over time. It will block the effect of opiates like heroin or hydrocodone. There is some abuse potential, but this medication is generally safe if taken as prescribed. The naloxone is inactive unless the drug is injected (a way to abuse the medication), and the activation blocks the medication from its partial-agonist effect. Suboxone is used for detox from opiates and in some cases used for long-term treatment in opiate dependence. It can be useful in cases where there are repeated relapses or problems with opiate dependence associated with chronic pain. It has replaced methadone in many cases. Some opiate addicts use Suboxone as a way to continue their opiate abuse; it allows them to detox themselves between opiate uses (e.g., prescription opiates or heroin) and be more comfortable when they can't score their drug.

Other strategies include Antabuse, which produces ill effects when you drink while taking it and has some similar reported effects with cocaine. Certain anticonvulsants like depakote or topiramate have reported benefits in reducing alcohol consumption.

## Medication Treatments for Psychiatric and Medical Comorbidity

Coexisting psychiatric illness such as depression, anxiety disorders, and personality disorders are common in addicted patients, including professionals (Rounsaville et al. 1998; Angres et al. 2003). Aggressive diagnosis and treatment of these conditions are essential for positive outcomes (So 2005). This holds true for medical comorbidity as well, especially chronic pain conditions that frequently co-occur.

## Depression

Depression commonly accompanies addiction. The challenge is to determine if it is a consequence of the addiction, which can often occur. If the depression was there prior to the onset of the addiction, or hung in there during periods of sustained abstinence and recovery, it may be separate from the addiction. Usually depressions that are secondary to the addiction go away after several days in recovery. If they hang on, treatment with an antidepressant may be necessary and poses no particular risk of abuse and may help even if the depression is secondary to the addiction. Mindfulness-based cognitive therapy for depression has also been presented as a novel approach for relapse prevention in substance abusers, and it may be helpful as an adjunctive option (Segal et al. 2001). In situations where it may be unclear if the depression is secondary to the addiction, we advise a drug holiday at some point to see if the antidepressant is still necessary. The following conditions can be more challenging.

## Anxiety Disorders

Anxiety is a very common symptom accompanying addiction. It can take many forms, but some common presentations are generalized anxiety and panic disorder (a more acute experience that can feel like a heart attack). Other presentations include social phobia and performance anxiety. These conditions can occur alone or together in clusters. Often, as with generalized anxiety and panic in particular, benzodiazepines like Xanax or Ativan are used. These are highly addicting, so alternatives need to be used to treat addicts. Like depression, many anxiety symptoms can be secondary to or made much worse by addiction and may stop or lessen considerably with time in recovery. When medication is called for, there are some nonaddicting options. A group of medications called beta blockers (like propranolol) may help. Gabapentin (Neurontin) can helpful in lower doses than usually prescribed. SSRIs such as Zoloft can be helpful for anxiety as well as depression. As mentioned earlier, acamprosate may help anxiety as well as craving for alcohol (Swift 2002).

**Sleep Problems**

Sleep problems are especially common in addiction. Again, the medications often used, like the hypnotics (e.g., Ambien) have significant abuse potential. There are different medications that can be helpful and nonaddicting, such as Neurontin, trazadone (an atypical antidepressant), and Seroquel (a newer antipsychotic). These uses are off-label (not specifically what the FDA approved them for) for these medications and typically prescribed in smaller doses than for on-label use and for a short period of time in hopes that sleep patterns are eventually reestablished in recovery. There are other strategies, including certain antidepressants like Remeron or the older tricyclics (e.g., Elavil) that can be tried. If there is a history of sleep problems predating the addiction or there is suspicion of some kind of sleep disorder (e.g., obstructive sleep apnea), a sleep study is advised (Kolla et al. 2011).

**ADD and ADHD**

Attention deficit disorder (ADD) or attention deficit hyperactivity disorder (ADHD) are not uncommon in addiction (Ohlmeier et al. 2008). An interesting study by Dr. Nora Volkow and her team recently noted that brain imaging (PET scans) supported evidence for disruption of the dopamine reward pathway associated with motivation in ADHD patients (Volkow et al., 2011). This of course would complicate issues where ADHD coincides with addiction, since motivation and reward are affected in both conditions. So, ADHD is important to diagnose and treat if it comes up in addiction. There are many treatment alternatives to potentially addicting stimulants for ADHD if it is present.

Effects of addiction also include inattention and impulsivity, and a period of time in sobriety should occur to see if this improves on its own. There are those that think that ADD, characterized by inattention with or without hyperactivity, always originates in childhood and may continue in adulthood, and others believe it can start in adulthood. In either case, while there is good evidence that stimulants like Adderall and Ritalin are quite useful in childhood (and can even reduce risk of addiction in adulthood (Compton and Volkow 2006), there are significant risks for dependence in using psychostimulants in adults with addiction, particularly among females (Lynskey and Hall 2001). We recommend a trial on atomoxitine (Strattera) or bupropion (Wellbutrin). Some serotonin norepinephrine reuptake inhibitors (SNRIs) can help with ADD as well. Recent evidence highlights that methylphenidate (MPH) as a first-line treatment in adults with ADHD is not effective in patients with comorbid addiction and can put addicts at risk for abuse (Koesters et al. 2009; Carpentier et al. 2005) Nonmedication interventions including meditation, neurofeedback, exercise, and cognitive behavioral therapy can also be very useful and have all demonstrated benefit in ADD.

# Chronic Pain

Chronic pain is extremely common in addiction, especially in opiate-dependent people. In some cases, the pain is an excuse for use; in others, the pain is real but may be exaggerated to justify use of opiates. In some cases, the pain can actually get worse from the chronic opiate use, something called "hyperalgesia" (Silverman 2009). In many cases the pain is real and so is the addiction. A condition called "pseudo addiction" happens when someone has real chronic pain and is dependent on opiates only because of the pain. Usually in pseudo addiction, there is no family history of addiction and there is no evidence of connection with the substance, such as a rewarding experience, that transcends pain relief (Dodrill et al. 2011).

There needs to be a careful workup to determine the origin of the pain often with a qualified pain specialist who understands addiction. In cases where there appears to be a legitimate source of pain, nonopiate approaches must be tried. Since low back pain is the most common chronic pain presentation, the use of nerve blocks or spinal cord stimulators should be investigated along with conservative medication management with muscle relaxants (which have some abuse potential over time), nonsteroidals (e.g., Celebrex), and Neurontin. Physical therapy is usually a critical long-term strategy as well. These approaches are useful with many musculoskeletal conditions where surgery may not be an option (Dodrill et al. 2011). In cases where there is an established need for narcotic analgesia, Suboxone may be a useful and safer pain management strategy (Heit and Gourlay 2008).

We have seen a number of true chronic pain conditions improve dramatically with a strong recovery that incorporates a healthy lifestyle—in other words, a positive sobriety. We have also instituted acupuncture and cold laser therapy and are seeing good responses in some of our patients.

**Plainly Stated:**

**Medications are often necessary for the reduction of craving, to block the effects of substances (to reduce potential for relapse), or to treat coexisting conditions like depression or anxiety. They may be necessary for the short term or longer, depending on the individual. In the case of substance blockers or anticraving medications, use may be necessary for several months to buy time until recovery is firmly established. Some of the more challenging coexisting conditions include chronic pain, attention deficit disorder, and sleep problems. These conditions are often treated with potentially addicting medications but can be managed well without them.**

## *PERSONAL PERSPECTIVE*

*When I first entered treatment in 1982, I struggled with guilt and shame. As a psychiatrist, I was trained to see addiction as a symptom of something else, such as depression or a personality disorder. This was the understanding of the day in the scientific and psychiatric community. Today this community fully embraces the disease model. My professional rejection of the disease model fueled my personal belief that I was defective and even weak willed. I can remember the day I heard the Disease of Chemical Dependency lecture given by the pioneer in addiction medicine, Doug Talbott, MD. It felt as if a weight had been lifted off my shoulders. I finally understood why I did what I did. It did not free me of the responsibility for my recovery, but it helped me get past an often paralyzing self-condemnation.*

DHA

# 3. Psychosocial Treatment: Software Interventions

Substance abuse negatively impacts public safety, reduces workers' productivity, and contributes to higher health care costs, premature deaths, and disability for millions of Americans (Hughes 2001). Despite this massive health problem, only a fraction of affected people get the help they need. A report released in September 2007 by the Substance Abuse and Mental Health Services Administration (SAMHSA) shows that in 2006, 23.6 million people aged twelve or older (9.6 percent of the population) required treatment for alcohol or drug problems, with only 2.5 million receiving the help (American Society of Addiction 2007). Even fewer get the treatment that works the best: psychosocial treatment.

The addicted brain struggling with deficits in reward, learning and memory, motivation, and decision making requires a comprehensive treatment approach. Physical, psychosocial, spiritual, and in many cases pharmacological interventions are necessary in treating addicted individuals. The disease model of addiction has promoted a number of effective pharmacological approaches to addiction; however, nonpharmacotherapeutic interventions are necessary and ultimately the most effective for long-term recovery.

As mentioned earlier, most individuals in early recovery benefit from treatment along with a therapeutic community, the implementation of nonchemical coping skills, and the fellowship of AA (Maxwell 1984). These interventions assist the addict in adopting more adaptive ways to create reward, improve decision making and motivation, and establish new memories. The nonpharmacotherapeutic strategies are powerful enough to create new connections between neurons, or neurogenesis. This can be likened to "software" approaches that change the hardware of the brain, as opposed to only looking at direct hardware approaches, like medication management or some form of neuromodulation, as mentioned previously. In many cases, however, the addict needs both. The path to recovery must be multifaceted to be successful.

## Positive Sobriety

### The Growth Cycle of Recovery

- Positive Sobriety
- Abstinence Based Treatment (Running on Empty)
- Abstinence Alone / Back to 2 Quarts Low — *Motivation*
- Changing Behavior & Thinking / Insight & Bonding (Group, Community, AA) — *Learning and Memory*
- Spiritual Program (e.g. Meditation) / Diet, Exercise — *Reward*
- Psychological, Emotional & Neurochemical Balance — *Decision Making*
- Maintenance Program (Recovery Counter Culture)

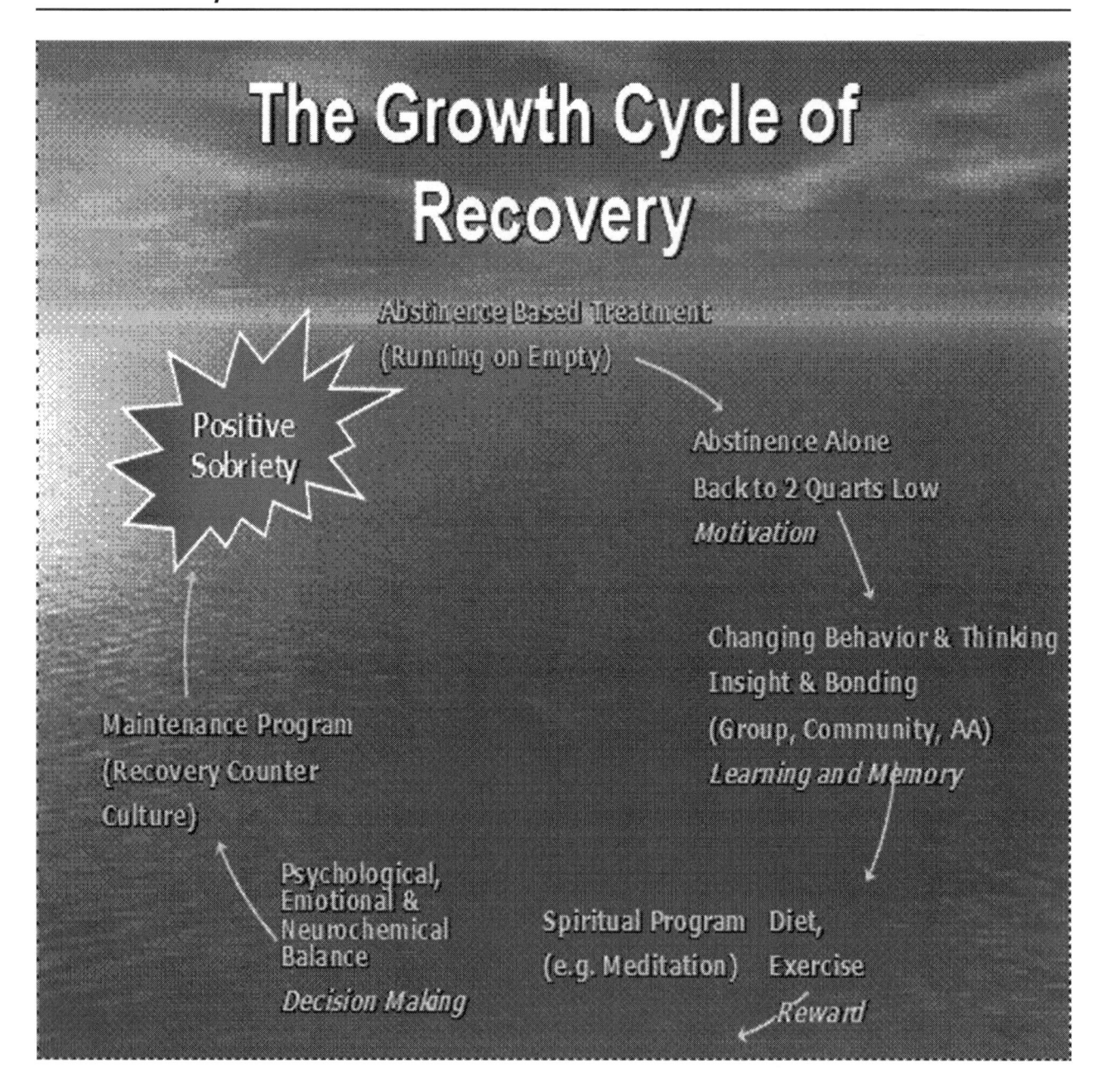

Figure 2: The above figure outlines how the disease model informs and guides the treatment process, moving from abstinence to positive sobriety through changing behavior, thinking, relationships, lifestyle, and ultimately neuronal pathways. This also correlates to enhancements in reward, learning and memory, motivation, and decision making.

## Our Treatment Structure

In the early 1940s, attempts were made to have AA partner with treatment programs, such as Wilmer hospital in Minnesota. Eventually, AA recognized the need for separation from the treatment programs within hospital systems. However, the philosophy of AA became integrated into the treatment process, revolutionizing treatment approaches and outcomes for generations. Pioneer House was the first treatment program in Minnesota to base its three-week residential program on the philosophy of Alcoholics Anonymous. This was called the Minnesota Model (White 1998). The program pioneered a treatment approach that incorporated twelve-step principles and influences while maintaining autonomy and a degree of distance from AA. This model also embraced the concept that alcoholism is a disease, not a symptom of an underlying psychiatric illness.

Today, most abstinence-based programs like ours have evolved from this model and have become more inclusive of psychological and pharmacological strategies. This model also has a rich history of utilizing a holistic and integrative approach to alcoholism and other addictions. This approach centers on a multidisciplinary team that includes recovering alcoholics and integrates the tenets of AA into the treatment process. Since the AA program has an emphasis on the spiritual aspects of recovery, AA has become an essential element of holistic treatment. The Minnesota Model lends itself to recovery because of a legacy that began with the advent of twelve-step recovery programs such as Alcoholics Anonymous, which began in 1935 (Spicer 1993; Anderson 1981; Laundergan 1982). According to Damian McElrath, as described in the *Journal of Psychoactive Drugs* (1997), AA contributed the following to the Minnesota Model: 1) the knowledge or belief that alcohol is a physical, mental, and spiritual illness; 2) the idea that the twelve steps outline the problem, solution, and the spiritual exercises needed to live in the solution; and 3) the understanding that fellowship and recovery takes place with one alcoholic talking to another.

Khantzian and Mack (1994) have reinforced the importance of the psychosocial support of a therapeutic community in the treatment of addictions. They state, "Alcohol and drug dependence are the result of complex interactions of biological, psychological, and cultural factors; yet, the most promising and successful interventions in these disorders are psychosocial in nature." Although AA and treatment separated rather early in the process, the connection between them remains vital for everyone who subscribes, in some form, to this model. Involvement in this model of treatment with aftercare and ongoing AA involvement has shown positive results (Project Match Research Group, 1997).

The structure of our program includes psychosocial support in a therapeutic community—that ability for support from other addicts and alcoholics within the framework of a day hospital setting—supplemented by a peer-supported independent living program (ILP). Our structure is derived from the Minnesota Model and one that Doug Talbott, MD, pioneered in the mid-1970s. The Talbott model is a four-month model that was primarily designed for the addicted health care professional. The first month was a residential experience after which the patient moved into independent living and spent a month in a day hospital setting then worked for the last two months as a health care professional in an addiction-related program in the community (e.g., Salvation Army Addiction Program) while remaining in the ILP. This last two months of step-down work was referred to as "placement," which this manual explains later on.

Over the years here in Chicago, we have streamlined the program to be more economically feasible and individualized but to still have the necessary clinical impact. In our book *Healing the Healer* and in more recent outcome studies (see appendix A), we established that we had comparable outcomes to the longer Talbott program. If our patients need an inpatient stay, it is typically for detox and stabilization done in a typically briefer period of a few days. Our length of stay averages eight weeks, with our step-down phase using the volunteerism program and placing the patient in a more advanced role within our program instead of in practice as a health care professional outside of our setting. This allows us to have more contact with the patient and enables us to have this important placement phase available to our non-health care professionals. This structure is not for everyone, as some patients need longer stays in an extended residential setting. We try to individualize our recommendations for treatment and to avoid a one-size-fits-all mind-set.

The modalities described in this chapter delineate our treatment approach within the structure we embrace. That structure includes two to four weeks in a day hospital setting with most living in the ILP. Step-down, or "placement," into the Intensive Outpatient (IOP) component following the patient's time in the day hospital allows the patient to continue in the critical morning small group process and engagement in the larger therapeutic community while having more time in the afternoons for individual needs like volunteerism and individual therapy. Nightly AA meetings during the week and at least one meeting a day on weekends is required.

### Alternative Option

Going through an intensive treatment program that includes the elements that this chapter describes is what we think is the best option for most addicts. But for many, this is not possible. Working a strong twelve-step program, often in conjunction with a skilled therapist who understands addiction, can work well for some. There are also excellent public and Veterans' Affairs programs that incorporate these essential treatment elements (see appendix C).

*PERSONAL PERSPECTIVE:*

*Going through treatment (in a very similar program to what I am running now) in 1982 saved my life, pure and simple.*

DHA

## A) Individualized Treatment Planning and Individual Therapy

The initial assessment allows us to determine the needs of each patient. This includes determining the need for hospitalization and whether our program is a therapeutic fit. Some patients may need more structure, like a residential experience, or less, like an evening outpatient program. We follow the ASAM patient placement criteria but recognize the special needs of some of our patients: for example, our health care professionals, who may need to be out of the workplace for a period of time for their own and their patients' protection. We also evaluate (sometimes on an ongoing basis) whether the ILP is viable, as some patients may need to commute. This can be the case if there are child care issues or if patients have certain necessary supports in the home. In any case, all patients, whether commuting to the program or living in the ILP, participate in the social support functions that happen around the ILP after hours and on weekends, as outlined later.

In the program, each patient is assigned a primary counselor with whom they work both individually and in small groups. This way the counselor knows the patient both in a group setting as well as individually. By virtue of this knowledge, along with additional information from history, family, and psychological testing, including the TCI self-reports, the individual therapist can create a treatment plan that relates to the unique individual needs of each patient.

As each of the three elements (the psychological, environmental, and biological) contributes in varying degrees to addiction and all illnesses, in order for any treatment to be fully effective, each element needs to be addressed. The psychological element is addressed in the small group experience, the larger therapeutic community, AA and didactic parts of the program, and individually with the primary counselor.

A recent review of the literature about the quality of clinicians and substance use disorder treatment outcomes highlights the importance of the individual impact of clinicians on their patients. Evidence suggests that clinicians are a key factor in influencing treatment outcome and retention. Use of written treatment protocols is noted to increase overall patient outcomes and to reduce variance by clinicians (Najavits et al. 2000). We have been fortunate to have highly skilled, compassionate, and committed primary counselors in our program.

Incorporating individual therapy into our treatment regime is an effective means to address those underlying psychological issues for some of our patients. Our preference is that, at least initially, the patient connect with the program in the first two to four weeks of day hospital before engaging in individual work. As the patient steps down to an intensive day outpatient setting, they will have more time to see an individual therapist for their special needs (for example, trauma work). Individual work does happen with the primary counselor, but sometimes more is needed. Most patients are recommended to individual therapy after they complete treatment. We have been impressed with the benefits of cognitive behavioral therapy (CBT).CBT addresses the negative self-talk and negative core beliefs that have been present in so many of our patients. CBT has been an effective treatment for many conditions, including depression, anxiety disorders, and addiction (when used as an adjunct to a treatment program regimen). In fact, many patients need to address their negative self-talk before they can effectively use meditation as a way to observe these thought patterns.

**Alternative Option**

There are many outstanding therapists in the community that can assess and help treat addicts. See appendix C for links.

*PERSONAL PERSPECTIVE*

*I will always remember my primary counselor, Wade Hopkins, from my treatment experience. Now deceased, Wade was a warm and wise and caring therapist. We met at intervals throughout the treatment process, and he would help guide me in various ways, sometimes sharing from his own experience. His help was a very important counterpoint to the group and therapeutic community and other aspects of treatment for me.*

*I recall in particular when he described his own experience of having a place where he could go to commune with nature and get out of the rat race of everyday life. Over the years, I have taken that advice to heart and have been able to take my family to a hilly area on the Illinois-Iowa border that allows for communing with the beauty of nature. This has helped shape not only my own life but our family's life in a very positive way.*

*DHA*

# B) Small Group Therapy

We believe the small group process is the most important component of any addiction treatment experience.

There is no one-size-fits-all approach to the treatment of addiction, although group therapy is one of the best therapies for those in recovery. The benefits of group therapy that have been noted are learning that others share similar issues and problems, the opportunity to see and learn from others who are at different stages in recovery, the sharing of individual problems with the group and receiving mutual feedback, the opportunity to improve social interactions, and the introduction to a recovery community. Group therapy has been regarded as both effective in the treatment of substance use disorders as well as being an economy of scale. As such, group therapy is regarded as a source of powerful curative forces not always experienced in individual therapy. The engagement of therapeutic forces in group therapy sessions (e.g., affiliation, support, and peer confrontation) enable patients to bond within a culture of recovery. Additionally, since addiction is often accompanied by depression, isolation, and shame, the group modality has great effectiveness in addressing these issues. Addiction therapy groups also help foster healthy attachments, provide positive peer reinforcement, act as a forum for self-expression, and teach new social skills. These positive effects have been associated with greater likelihood of commitment to abstinence than through individual therapy (SAMHSA 2005)

Two assignments are proposed to help facilitate connection with yourself and ultimately the small group. One is called "How It Was" and encourages the addict to explore and organize in writing an autobiography It can be helpful to refer to your Temperament and Character Inventory scores to identify character strengths and weaknesses when composing this assignment. Following "How It Was" is "How It Will Be," which is designed as a means to practice optimism, effort, and intention. The "How It Will Be" exercise provides the addict with an opportunity to directly confront the future and describe how things will be different than they were in the past when the addiction was prominent. It provides specific goals and aspirations to work toward and look forward to in the long term.

In addition to the written assignments, small group therapy provides a structured format for addicts to address any issues or problems that affect recovery in an environment that allows for open discussion and feedback. Through the small group process, denial is confronted and self-awareness promoted by sharing experiences, feelings, and beliefs. Behaviors that are conducive to recovery are explored and practiced while detrimental behaviors and beliefs are confronted. Addicts practice self-disclosure in a supportive environment to promote direct and honest communication and to prepare them for participation in twelve-step recovery groups. The process of reciprocal, supportive communication fostered within the small group reduces the guilt, shame, isolation, and alienation often felt by addicts. Within the community, many individual therapists run small groups or can direct you to them. Heinz Kohut spoke of a "room full of mirrors" to describe group therapy: it is a place where people can see themselves in others.

**Alternative Options**

Some therapists in the community run small groups that focus on addiction and recovery.

*PERSONAL PERSPECTIVE*

*I was very depressed early on in treatment. I can remember sitting in small group wondering why anyone would talk at all. What possible good would talking with these people ever do? Give me meds, for God's sake! After several weeks I was in a group where one group member was confronting another about his hopelessness and inactivity. All of a sudden I spoke up and joined in the confrontation. The group members were shocked. This was the first time I had said anything beyond my name or monosyllabic grunts in group. I eventually realized I was confronting my own hopelessness and inactivity. Truly, an epiphany occurred in group that day. My depression spontaneously remitted, as did my inactivity, from that group interaction. I will always marvel at the power of the group process.*

*DHA*

## Specialty Groups

### Caduceus group

The Caduceus group meets weekly and provides a forum for licensed and other professionals to specifically address work-related issues, including return-to-work plans. There is often shame about the interface of addiction and occupation and certain risks associated with many jobs (e.g., a nurse going back to dispensing narcotics or a lawyer returning to a workplace that celebrates drinking). This group of peers can be a powerful tool in paving the way to a supportive work environment. Health care professionals, when treated appropriately in a professionals program with extended aftercare and joint monitoring with a state professional health program, have excellent outcomes. Studies have shown upwards of 73 percent of these patients had two or more years of continuous sobriety (see Angres and Dupont, and our study in appendix A).

### AID group

The weekly group for addiction interactive disorder (AID) is a safe place for those individuals with AID issues like sexual compulsivity, compulsive eating, or compulsive gambling can be with others who have these same coexisting problems. Led by a clinician credentialed in this area, the AID group provides direction in recovery for these specific issues.

### Comorbidity group

Patients who have comorbid conditions like depression or anxiety can access a weekly group that specifically works with these conditions. Here patients can freely address these issues as a priority within a peer group setting run by a staff person with expertise in these conditions.

### Alternative Options

There are many specialty groups available, including twelve-step groups that work with comorbidity or AID issues. Also, there are peer support groups all over the country. For Caduceus support, there are state medical society or board-sponsored advocacy groups called professionals' health programs (PHPs) and similar programs for other groups (like the Lawyers' Assistance Programs). See the appendix B.

# C) Therapeutic Community

In our professionals program, most patients live in apartments we provide and externally supervise, called the Independent Living Program (ILP). These living arrangements create small family units separated by gender. The patients spend the day at the partial program then return to the ILP. They usually have dinner together before going to an AA or other twelve-step meeting in small groups. They also help each other with rides and orienting new patients. Sometimes a patient who is struggling or new in the program is supported by others in the community. This is referred to as "shadowing." There are also community activities like the Thursday all-community dinner and the Sunday outing. The patients learn to support each other and prioritize recovery as a value. From serious talks to sober fun, this aspect of the program is a powerful therapeutic experience.

The National Institute for Drug Abuse (NIDA), an affiliate of the National Institutes of Health (NIH), defines the therapeutic community (TC) as a residential setting that uses a hierarchical model of treatment reflecting increased levels of personal and social responsibility (2002). Peer influence is used in a variety of group processes to help patients progress through treatment. TCs employ the "community as method" approach to treatment; namely, the treatment staff and patients both contribute to change with the shared goal of individual and group well-being and sobriety. TC members interact in structured and unstructured ways to influence the behaviour's, attitudes, and perceptions that accompany drug use. As well as employing the community, the TC theory also emphasizes the importance of the self (self-help) as the primary agent of change. The concept, "mutual self-help" refers to patients' assuming partial responsibility for the recovery of their peers, which also aids in a patient's own treatment (De Leon 2000).

In such a community, modeling more adaptive behaviours by senior patients and an overall expectation of abstinence and compliance with the rules of the program create a safe setting for recovery from addiction. These expectations are complemented by the camaraderie and empathy of the other patients in the community and enhance the motivation and compliance of addicts to seek recovery. In his article, "AA and the Governance of Self," John Mack (1981) emphasized the importance of community in recovery. He described self-governance as "the sense of being and the power to be in charge of oneself as one of the most highly valued of human functions" (p. 133). However, he also pointed out that the self never functions as a solitary entity. In this sense, self-governance allows for sharing control or responsibility with other individuals or groups. The result is self-governance supported by mutual help. The NIDA has conducted studies on treatment programs that utilize the therapeutic community model and has found that patients who have successfully completed treatment in a TC have lower levels of drug use, unemployment, criminal behaviour, and depression indicators than before treatment (NIDA 2002).

There is also an added treatment phase called mirror image therapy that is often used in professionals programs. This involves the professional acting in a senior patient role with tasks such as helping the treatment staff with orienting and otherwise assisting newer patients. We call mirror image therapy "shadowing" in our program. The twelve steps and twelve traditions observe how important it is for addicts to see others in the program confront and transcend their pain and negativity because these acts provide a tangible example of optimism in action. Mirror imaging hopefully allows the senior patient to see themselves in others, while the junior patient has a model of success to strive for, creating empathy and self-insight. It additionally provides a transition at the end of treatment that facilitates the senior patient in their return to work as a helping professional.

**Alternative Option**

There are a number of living environments for recovering people. Specifically, there are halfway houses, which are typically the most restrictive, three-quarter-way houses that are less restrictive, and finally Oxford Houses, in which recovering people live together. The appendix B lists ways one can access these various living environments. Many do require a period of sobriety prior to entrance; however, most do not require being in a treatment experience prior to entry.

### *PERSONAL PERSPECTIVE*

*Living with other men in the Independent Living Program was one of the most important elements of my program. The epiphany that occurred that day in small group, as stated earlier, carried over to the apartment living situation. I recall very well to this day the evening of that small group process: it was my turn to prepare dinner for my apartment mates that evening. Prior to that group experience, I was quiet and isolative and took no joy in any of the community activities, including the meal preparation. In my program then, as is the case in our program now, having a communal dinner bonded us as a family. I can remember peeling potatoes and feeling a sense of connection and purpose and meaning in that humble act. I recognize that my ability to really be with others who were on the same path was a unique gift.* **DHA**

## D) Family Program

The first chance for patients to make amends is often to family and loved ones. A sense of relief is the most prevalent feeling family members experience when the addict/alcoholic commits to enter treatment and begin recovery. As treatment progresses, the family is invited to participate in the program. Loved ones are strongly encouraged to engage in the formal and social aspects of the treatment program, to attend Al-Anon or other twelve-step support groups and, if necessary, continue or begin individual psychotherapy for support.

The most important aspect of family involvement in a professional's treatment program is Family Week. Family Week lasts three days and consists of an educational component combined with multifamily group therapy. The educational aspect often includes an emphasis on the most recent evidence-based scientific data that supports the disease model of addiction along with practical advice for family, especially regarding relapse prevention. The education also prepares loved ones for the multifamily component of the program. Multifamily group therapy consists of family and loved ones plus patients, each presenting written homework assignments to one another in a small group led by a counselor. The effectiveness of this approach is the bonding and similarities the participants experience, and increased communication and insight for all group members.

An alternative option for those loved ones that are unable to attend a three-day Family Week is Monday of Family Week for education only. However, the three-day program is the preferred choice.

Prior to Family Week, the patient and their loved ones are invited to attend an hour-long family session that includes the patient, their loved ones, and both the primary counselor and the family therapist. This session is an opportunity to gather insight about the patient from their loved ones with the patient present and gives family members an opportunity to have their thoughts and feelings heard and questions answered. Personal information about the patient is not shared with loved ones without the patient's consent; therefore, the session is an important time to begin to integrate the family into the recovery program. Additionally, the patients feel more secure and supported knowing they are a part of the information gathering. The session is typically scheduled within the first three weeks of treatment, and Family Week is scheduled close to the patient's discharge date.

Al-Anon is a twelve-step approach for family members, and like Alcoholics Anonymous and other twelve-step recovery programs, its meetings are numerous and easily accessible. Al-Anon is strongly encouraged for all loved ones for support and personal recovery.

There is also a Support Group for Significant Others that meets every Tuesday evening at the program. A therapist facilitates this group. It is confidential, and it is complimentary. The aftercare program meets at the same time and place, making it conducive for loved ones and patients to continue the connection to the program after treatment together. The Significant Others group is available to loved ones for two years.

Last, the patients host two recovery-oriented social events each week that are open to loved ones. There is a Thursday evening community dinner and open AA meeting at the apartments, and a Sunday afternoon event.

*Family involvement will positively impact long-term recovery and healing in the family.*

## Alternative Option

Family members and loved ones of addicts and alcoholics need to recover from the adverse effects of the disease too. Most people benefit from Al-Anon, Families Anonymous, Codependents Anonymous, or Alateen, which are easily accessible, free, and inclusive settings. Psychotherapy and programs such as Onsite (see appendix B) are also helpful but require financial resources.

**Positive Sobriety**

*PERSONAL PERSPECIVE:*

*My family and significant other wanted to support me but had no idea about the disease and the recovery process. Going through the family program was of critical importance for them and for me.*

*DHA*

## E) Twelve-Step Programs

Alcoholics Anonymous (AA) is the most widely used resource for alcoholism and addiction recovery by addicts and treatment programs. In the professionals program, we require patients to attend daily twelve-step meetings and get a temporary sponsor. AA meeting attendance is positively associated with long-term abstinence (Kaskutas 2005; Hoffman et al. 1983; Hoffman and Kaplan 1991; Hoffman and Miller 1992).

Twelve-step recovery is a spiritually based program that supports a healthier relationship with self, others, and ultimately a higher power. You may notice that the Character scales of the TCI closely resemble promotion of a healthier relationship with self, others, and the transcendent as a path to well-being. AA is also a practical program that identifies three key components for sobriety:

1) What is the problem?

2) What is the solution?

3) What is the action needed to recover?

The problem is the addiction. The beginning of that search for the solution is reflected in the twelve steps of AA. The action needed to recover is accomplished through adhering to a twelve-step program. AA's twelve steps (Alcoholics Anonymous 1976) are spiritually based principles designed to foster a way of life that is happy and successful in the absence of substance use. The addict is to "work the steps" in a progression. They are as follows:

1) We admitted that we were powerless over alcohol—that our lives had become unmanageable.

2) Came to believe that a power greater than ourselves could restore us to sanity.

3) Made a decision to turn our will and our lives over to the care of God *as we understood Him.*

4) Made a searching and fearless moral inventory of ourselves.

5) Admitted to God, ourselves, and to another human being the exact nature of our wrongs.

6) Were entirely ready to have God remove all these defects of character.

7) Humbly asked Him to remove our shortcomings.

8) Made a list of all persons we had harmed and became willing to make amends to them all.

9) Made direct amends to such people wherever possible, except when to do so would injure them or others.

10) Continued to take personal inventory, and when we were wrong promptly admitted it.

11) Sought through prayer and meditation to improve our conscious contact with God as we understood Him, praying for knowledge of His will for us and the power to carry that out.

12) Having had a spiritual awakening as the result of these steps, we tried to carry this message to alcoholics and to practice these principles in all our affairs.

From the twelve steps, twelve promises have evolved (Alcoholics Anonymous 1953). These twelve promises expand the message of the twelve steps and provide a positive outlook on the future as a result of working the twelve steps and adopting them as a script for life. They are as follows:

1) We are going to know a new freedom and a new happiness.

2) We will not regret the past nor wish to shut the door on it.

3) We will comprehend the word serenity.

4) We will know peace.

5) No matter how far down the scale we have gone, we will see how our experience can benefit others.

6) That feeling of uselessness and self-pity will disappear.

7) We will lose interest in selfish things and gain interest in our fellows.

8) Self-seeking will slip away.

9) Our whole attitude and outlook on life will change.

10) Fear of people and economic insecurity will leave us.

11) We will intuitively know how to handle situations which used to baffle us.

12) We will suddenly realize that God is doing for us what we could not do for ourselves.

You will notice how similar these twelve promises are to the literature of positive psychology described throughout this book. The combination of the tenets of AA with the philosophy of positive psychology and with elements of your unique personality informs the idea of creating a positive sobriety. We require attendance at twelve-step meetings in our program.

**Alternative Option**

One of the great gifts of Alcoholics Anonymous and other twelve-step recovery programs is their availability. Twelve-step recovery has been the bedrock for so many addicts and their ability to be in recovery. There are meetings all over the world and now on the Internet as well. Appendix C of this book lists ways to contact any number of twelve-step recovery programs. For some, SMART Recovery is an alternative self-help organization that takes a less spiritual and more directive, rational approach to recovery. This may be an alternative to explore for those who struggle with AA for whatever reason. There is evidence that an increasing number of recovering people are actually going to both, finding them compatible.

*PERSONAL PERSPECTIVE*

*I will always remember my first meeting; this was directly prior to coming into a treatment program in 1982. This was what is called a speaker's meeting, in which someone shares for a good part of the meeting their own personal experience. I recall the speaker, Bob S., introducing himself: "Hi, I'm Bob. And I'm a grateful recovering addict and alcoholic." I was dumbfounded. I could not imagine how anyone could be grateful for being an addict. After many years of sobriety, I understand this very well today and have made it the underlying theme of this book: addiction with all its initial pleasure and eventual pain can be a path to well-being and happiness. This has certainly been the case in my life.*

DHA

# F) Volunteerism

According to Alfred Adler, the highly acclaimed and renowned father of the school of individual psychology, well-being is enhanced through social movement and positive associations made with others, termed *gemeinschaftsgefuhl*. This has been translated to mean "community feeling," or acting with regard to social interest. Intrinsically, we have a sense of obligation and responsibility to the general welfare of people, and by creating an empathetic, emotional bond with others, we can enact a sense of community that enables us to incorporate our individual sense of feeling to that of feeling at home in the world. In short, community feeling equals *volunteerism.*

Volunteers benefit society. They add to the quality and capacity of programs and services by providing enthusiasm, extra resources, and many times much needed skills. They supplement the normal workforce during times of crisis, especially when workload demands peak. Further, volunteers who are trained and experienced provide a ready pool of applicants for employment. So, what does volunteering have to do with sobriety and recovery? When we engage in volunteerism, it pulls us out of our normal calculating world of profit and loss. We get out of the control mode and into the communal cooperative sharing mode that is essential to becoming a whole human being. In this way, we integrate recovery with a holistic picture of health, one that is on the pathway to achieving not only sobriety, but *positive* sobriety.

Volunteerism is also a critical component to twelve-step recovery. Step twelve, "Having had a spiritual awakening as the result of these steps, we tried to carry this message to others and to practice these principles in all our affairs," evidences the mutual benefit of volunteerism for those in recovery and their communities. Giving back to the community by carrying the message enables the individual in recovery to reengage in society as an active member acting in its interest. Not only is volunteerism inspired by the twelfth step, but through its transformative personal process and focus on providing service and sustaining value, *volunteerism is an alternative to relapse.* Within the recovery community, volunteerism is present through the very existence of AA, NA, and other twelve-step groups. Activities such as helping set up for meetings, assisting in planning a recovery event, giving a formal lead, and taking on a sponsee are all illustrations of volunteerism at work to enhance sobriety. Volunteerism also continues the legacy of the Talbott model during the placement phase of treatment previously described.

In recognizing the link between community feeling, enhanced well-being, and sobriety, we have formally incorporated volunteerism into the Positive Sobriety program. As part of their overall treatment goals, patients are required to provide a minimum of two hours of volunteer services to the community per week. Upon arrival, patients are oriented to a number of potential volunteer opportunities as well as registered on a citywide registry of community service projects they can sign up for online (www.ChicagoCares.org). Senior members of the treatment community are paired with new members to mentor in this process, and a community volunteerism coordinator is made available for assistance and support during scheduled office hours. A sign-up log is posted in a central location each week for patients to record and track their service hours, and service experiences are discussed and evaluated weekly by the treatment team. In addition, a volunteerism committee made up of an elected member of the treatment community, the community volunteerism coordinator, and several staff members of the treatment team meet on a regular basis to conduct continuous quality improvement efforts of the volunteerism program and to engage in feedback sessions with community partners.

## Positive Sobriety

We believe treatment provides an opportunity to expand the definition of what is commonly thought of as volunteerism and to find the setting that is right for each individual in the long term. Whatever activity sticks with an individual, whether walking dogs for a local shelter, taking a pro bono client in the professional sector, tutoring a high school student for the GED, sorting clothes at a thrift store, helping with a church bake sale, or bringing meals to a senior citizen in need, continued engagement will foster well-being manifested in positive sobriety.

**Alternative Options**

See appendix B for the many ways you can volunteer in the community.

*PERSONAL PERSPECTIVE:*

*Going through placement in treatment then later volunteering in twelve-step recovery (including sponsoring people) demonstrated the power of volunteering. My wife and I have continued to volunteer over the years.*

*DHA*

# G) Diet and Exercise

### Diet

Foods have been used as nourishment as well as cures for a plethora of ailments throughout history in all cultures. Unfortunately, in our current fast-paced, grab-and-go culture, the vital role nutrition plays in our vitality is lost to trans fats and over processed packaged foods. Part of living a healthy lifestyle within the goal of positive sobriety includes extending the effort into making sound dietary choices. Watching what you eat and following a balanced diet contributes to overall health and works against the development of diseases such as diabetes, heart disease, and cancers. Bad dietary habits can contribute to emotional disorders and difficulties in concentration. Human nutrition is complex, and what constitutes a "healthy diet" may vary widely depending on genetic, environmental, and individual health factors.

Neurotransmitter dysregulation, particularly of dopamine, serotonin, and glutamate, can result from not eating well (not eating enough or not eating the right foods), meaning that the body is not making enough of these chemicals to effectively ward off symptoms of depression and anxiety. In his book "The Dopamine Diet" Dr. Ken Blum outlines the importance of diet to augment dopamine in the addict.

Skipping meals can also have the effect of making blood sugar fall too low. Eating starchy, sugary foods, or simple carbohydrates (e.g., white bread and pastries), can spike blood sugar levels too high. Such extreme rises and falls of blood sugar affect mood states, resulting in greater negative mood states such as irritability, forgetfulness, sadness, and worry. For mental well-being, blood sugar needs to be kept steady by not skipping meals and instead eating smaller meals and healthy snacks throughout the day. In order to feel your best, you cannot starve your brain. The brain is made up of foods, and eating the right foods is the foundation for good health. A weight-loss plan that simply cuts fat and calories is a recipe for failure. Without natural mood boosters in the diet (e.g., magnesium, vitamin B12, and conjugated linoleic acid), feelings of happiness are less likely to be experienced. Further, following an extremely low-fat diet is countereffective. The body needs some healthy fats to promote brain function and positive mood states. Eating healthy monounsaturated fats (e.g., from olive oil, fatty fish) instead of saturated fats (e.g., from butter, fast foods) helps facilitate both brain functioning and happiness. Fruits and vegetables rich in vitamin B6, folic acid, vitamin C, and zinc also help manufacture serotonin, the neurotransmitter that regulates not only mood, but also sleep and appetite. It is suggested that a diet higher in complex carbohydrates as found in fruits and vegetables and lower in sodium, sugar, and saturated fat is conducive to physical and emotional well-being. Diet plans such as the ones found in Graham and Ramsey's 2011 book *The Happiness Diet* or Vogel and Lehr's 2008 book *The Pritikin Edge* show the integration of mindful eating for health and happiness and also allow for customized plans for holistic well-being.

**Exercise**

Exercise is proven therapy for depression and anxiety and also very helpful in improving cognition and decision making. Most notably, exercise is an effective and nonchemical way to cause the release of serotonin and dopamine—neurochemicals associated with good feelings. Persistence in an exercise regime, particularly one aerobic in nature, is related with an increase in the enzymes that make dopamine, an increase in the mechanisms of the brain that make use of dopamine, and an increase in levels of serotonin. Therefore, not only are you training your body during exercise, but you are also training your brain. Try it—next time you're feeling down, try taking a brisk twenty- or thirty-minute walk. Notice how you feel before you leave, then how you feel when you get back home. Are there any differences in your mood?

Research (Putnam 2001) suggests that not only does exercise improve mood, but it can also improve attention, memory, and impulse control. These cognitive abilities are important when considering your return to the workplace as well as your reintegration from a structured environment such as the treatment community to your everyday life. Making exercise a part of your routine will give you a healthy way to take charge of your own happiness, from a neurochemical perspective.

Exercise has also been shown to have a positive impact on the treatment and prevention of substance use disorders. Exercise increases dopamine levels in the brain (Hattori et al. 1994), which has been shown to be dysregulated in addictions, therefore helping to modulate this neurotransmitter. Emerging evidence from animal and human studies shows that exercise may be useful in the treatment and prevention of substance use disorders (Thanos et al. 2010; Brown et al. 2010; Buchowski et al. 2011). Further, exercise has been shown to have positive effects on reducing tobacco cravings, withdrawal symptoms, and smoking-related behaviors (Taylor et al. 2007). Exercise also reduces anxiety. We have long known that a state of anxiety has been shown to acutely diminish after individual episodes of exercise (Raglin and Morgan 1987). A majority of studies have suggested the benefit of exercise in reducing stress-related symptoms across a variety of study populations, including nonclinical, clinical, and medically compromised adult populations (Lion 1978; Bahrke and Morgan 1978; Blumenthal et al. 1982; Prossner et al. 1981). Newer research has shown that even a short, two-week exercise intervention has significant effects on reducing anxiety sensitivity relative to a control group. This effect mediated the benefits of exercise on negative-affect states inducing anxious and depressed moods (Smits et al. 2008). Studies have also documented strong evidence for the general health benefits of regular moderate physical activity, citing the following improvements: lower risks of early death from chronic lifestyle diseases (heart disease, type II diabetes, stroke, high blood pressure, adverse blood lipid profile, metabolic syndrome, colon cancer, breast cancer), prevention of weight gain, weight loss when combined with diet interventions, improved cardiorespiratory and muscular fitness, improved cognition, and reduced depression (Leavitt 2008).

Exercise is particularly effective for the treatment of psychiatric conditions and symptoms. Aerobic exercise interventions are useful in the treatment of a wide range of psychiatric conditions, including anxiety and depression, and as an adjunctive treatment for certain physical health problems. Aerobic exercise interventions have been clinically shown to reduce depressive symptoms in both inpatient and outpatient settings (e.g., Dunn et al. 2005; Trivedi et al. 2006; Blumenthal et al. 1999). Exercise has been further found to have benefits when compared to medication, group therapy, and cognitive-behavioral therapy. A review of literature also found that exercise has the effect of reducing depressive and anxiety symptoms as well as increasing positive mood states, regardless of population (Byrne and Byrne 1993).

In regards to improvements in cognition, met analyses of randomized, controlled trials confirm that normal and cognitively impaired adults derive cognitive benefits from physical exercise (Etnier et al. 2006; Heyn et al. 2004; Angevaren et al. 2008). Improvements are the greatest for executive control processes (e.g., planning, scheduling, multitasking) for participants in combined strength- and aerobic-training regimens and when exercise duration is greater than thirty minutes (Colcombe and Kramer 2003). In these studies, improvements were also seen in motor and auditory functions, cognitive speed, and visual attention (Angevaren et al. 2008). After a full year of aerobic exercise, subjects of one study also demonstrated larger hippocampal volumes, the brain structure implicated in memory (Erikson et al. 2011). We have to remember the importance of cognition and memory in decision making and maintaining sobriety.

In a NIDA-funded study to characterize the effects of an aerobic- and resistance-exercise intervention (three days per week of exercise training) compared to health education in a population of chemically dependent individuals in a residential treatment center, the exercise group had improvements in their aerobic capacities, increases in chest and leg strength, decreases in relative body fat, improved endurance, improved reaction times, and overall declines in mood disturbances in both depression and anxiety states (Rawson et al. 2011). Finally, engaging in at least thirty minutes of exercise three times a week has been shown to be just as effective in treating mild or moderate depression as taking antidepressants. In one study, engaging in exercise at the public health dose of 17.5 kilocalories per kilogram per week was shown to reduce depressive symptoms by as much as 47 percent (Dunn et al. 2005).

**Alternative Option**

There are countless books and programs that are available for diet and nutrition. Some of what has been helpful for us is listed in appendix B.

*PERSONAL PERSPECTIVE*

*Although exercise had always been important for me, during my treatment experience, I recognized the benefit of a sustained and regular exercise program. This is something that has been an essential part of my recovery for the past twenty-seven years. I have also had struggles, as many addicts do, with eating patterns. In the last few years, I have found a program that is particularly beneficial. This program is called the Pritikin Program that has its base in Miami Beach, Florida (Vogel and Lehr 2008). Appendix B also outlines a way to contact this program and a book that represents their diet plan. This is a medically oriented and, in my mind, very sensible program that emphasizes low-salt, low-fat, and low-sugar meals. It also emphasizes what it describes as low-density calories that are found in fruits and vegetables and certain whole grains. I found that this diet actually was something that was easy to sustain in terms of a lifestyle and a way of eating. In addition to having a dramatic reduction in blood pressure, cholesterol, and triglycerides, I have also noticed a substantial reduction in my previous tendency to turn to food as a source of comfort or diversion.*

*DHA*

# H) Continuing Care

Long-term, intensive follow up is critical to a good outcome for addiction. Essential to a treatment program is aftercare. In our program, this is structured to be a two-year minimum experience that includes weekly professionally facilitated support and monitoring groups; expected attendance in twelve-step recovery programs (or alternative mutual support groups); random urine, blood, or hair analyses; and interval visits with the treatment physician. Random drug testing allows for our monitoring of the recovering individual and at the same time can be evidence that the recovering individual is demonstrating compliance with the abstinence agreement. This continuing care program also monitors compliance with other aspects of a continuing care plan, such as individual or marital counseling and engagement with a psychiatrist or primary care physician in a hospital, group practice, or licensing board when applicable. Much different from the small group process while a patient is within the treatment facility, aftercare groups primarily allow individuals who have completed the program to share their experiences in recovery on a regular basis with a group leader and other people in the aftercare program. This also gives the therapist an opportunity to get a sense of an individual's recovery by monitoring their progress and ultimately holding the individual accountable for their contract.

We have something that's called a Caduceus Contract, which outlines a patient's aftercare plan in detail. This would include the expectations as they may exist for work, family, and individual recovery; expectations for twelve-step recovery involvement with sponsorship; individual therapy; certain work restrictions; and a plan for inclusion of any other individuals or entities that would be part of the recovery process. This could include a state medical society assistance program monitoring entity and/or an individual in someone's work setting who would know about the addiction and support and help monitor an individual in a workplace setting. This is, of course, all done with the patient's written permission.

The continuing care strategies described above are usually available in a similar fashion for other professional groups. For example, lawyer assistance programs are widespread throughout the United States, and employee assistance programs often fulfill the same role as state medical society assistance programs. For highly safety-sensitive professionals, federal regulatory agencies are often involved in this monitoring role. An example of this is the Federal Aviation Administration, which helps monitor commercial airline pilots in recovery. This group in particular has extremely high compliance and recovery rates. Concomitant support and monitoring occurs for five or more years with state-sponsored monitoring programs.

**Alternative Option**

There are a number of monitoring programs that can be accessed. Often these programs will allow individuals who have not been formally treated in their programs to participate in their monitoring. Appendix B lists state agencies as well as other entities that can be accessed for the purpose of aftercare monitoring.

*PERSONAL PERSPECTIVE*

*I can recall going to several aftercare meetings after my initial treatment experience. After four or five aftercare meetings, I became somewhat bored with the process. The meetings were not nearly as dynamic as the small group psychotherapy had been during treatment. Some of the rigors of the aftercare Caduceus Contract and the overall monitoring program seemed almost judgmental and heavy-handed at times. However, upon completion of the aftercare, I recognized how important it was to have this process. As I entered into real life, it was essential for me to have the ability to be accountable to others, particularly during stressful and difficult times.*

*DHA*

# 4. Core Treatment Lectures and Workshops

Common elements surface in the treatment of addictions, and to maintain a holistic approach to addiction treatment, addressing these manifestations is important. The most common of these are denial, grief, intimacy, anger, nicotine, post-acute withdrawal syndrome, relapse, AA (1 and 2), shame and guilt, codependency, impact of addiction on the family, stages of change, and use of the *Know Yourself* DVD series. Each of these lectures and workshops were developed by the staff at our program named in each section.

## Denial

*Wally Cross RPH, MHS, CADC*

Defense mechanisms are strategies employed by the psyche to cope with reality, protect the self from anxiety, and maintain self-image. They are used by everyone throughout life and only become pathological when persistent use of a defense leads to maladaptive behavior patterns that compromise the physical or mental health of the person. They are broken down into four levels, with progression through to the fourth level indicating more mature psychological functioning. The more immature the defense mechanism as defined by how far it removes the person from reality, the more likely that the person will exhibit difficulty coping, which will translate into interpersonal difficulties in work and personal relationships (Firestone 1987). In this lecture, the concept of denial and other defenses commonly used by substance abusers are discussed. In particular, these defenses are:

1) Denial: maintaining something is not so that is in fact so; this also includes dishonesty. Denial is a level one defense, indicating the individual is the most removed from reality.

2) Blaming (projection): denying responsibility for one's actions and maintaining that the responsibility lies with someone or something else. The behavior is not denied, but the cause is externalized. Blaming/projection can be either a level two or level three defense, depending on how persecutory the blaming is. Generally, if the blaming is directed at another person, it is a lower level defense than blaming unnamed elements.

3) Diversion: changing the subject. A level two defense, typical for adolescents.

4) Hostility: becoming angry, irritable, or aggressive with the result of avoiding the issue by scaring people off—people will generally avoid bringing up the topic in the future for fear of further hostility. A level two defense, hostility can be expressed either overtly in acting out, or passively as passive-aggressiveness.

5) Minimizing: admitting to some degree that a problem exists, but in such a way that it appears less serious or significant than it actually is. This is between a level two and level three defense, depending on how removed from reality the person is.

6) Rationalization: offering alibis, excuses, justifications, and other explanations for behavior. The behavior is not denied, but an inaccurate explanation for its cause is given.

7) Intellectualization: avoiding emotional or personal awareness of the problem by generalizing it in an intellectual or theoretical way. Intellectualization and rationalization are level three defenses, working toward a more mature psychological representation. Although they are typified as neurotic, they are common in adults.

After a brief overview of these defenses, the class is divided into two groups who are then asked to create two skits each in which they incorporate the defenses. Each group then presents their skits to the other group, which is in charge of identifying the defenses being used in each skit. This learn-by-doing method is engaging and effective for the patients, often instigating recall by the patients of which of these defenses they used while active in their addiction. The patients have an opportunity to gain some insight and awareness into their past modes of coping and are able to identify actions as defenses that they may not have recognized in the past (Vaillant 1992).

# Grief

*Anthony Loeb, MA, CADC*

Feelings of isolation, inadequacy, and humiliation are endemic to a community seeking treatment for addiction. The cumulative pain—a history that can include futility and failure—may perpetuate feelings of intense grief that need exploration. The psychological pain may be intolerable, and all patients are in a grieving process whether they know it or not. Initially patients come to us with emotional lives that may be blunted and with a limited emotional repertoire, but gradually in our two-part seminar, patients identify and process core feelings of grief and loss.

The Kubler-Ross model (evolved since 1969) outlines five stages of grief:

1. Denial

2. Anger

3. Bargaining

4. Depression

5. Acceptance

While Kubler-Ross's work has become a classical reference, our experience has shown that the stages may not reveal themselves sequentially Our primary concern is to help people gain insight into past experience and to explore how current struggles may originate in formative feelings of loss, regret, and humiliation that, until explored and resolved, remain essential components of grief.

Our workshop is experiential. We are arranged in a tight circle of chairs to promote intimacy and closeness. Grief is a subjective experience, an existential entity, but gradually the sharing deepens and patients begin to identify core feelings of loss that may be teased out from experiences such as the death of a parent or the ambiguity in the words "loss of innocence."

Egendorf (1995) discusses the importance of acknowledging and validating individual experiences of suffering and the transformative process involved in the sharing of personal stories. By giving grief a voice, the connection to and acceptance of oneself is deepened. Grief, unattended and unresolved, may be transmuted into intolerable, debilitating shame. When a commonality of experience of a broken marriage, of a formidable parental conflict is sought and shared, there can be profound resolution and relief.

Within the workshop, mutuality and empathy deepens, and the grief begins to resolve in a kind of catharsis, tentatively experienced at first.

As part of our process, people are asked to bring a symbol, a tangible, visual representation of their grief. Examples from past workshops have included pictures of one's parents, a medical license, a whip meant to symbolize the punishment imposed on a child, a lit candle that when extinguished was meant to represent one's loss of innocence.

In our work collectively, patients begin the process of reconnecting to their own histories and are able to find dignity and compassion and reaffirmation in their shared experience of loss.

# Anger

*Stephanie Bologeorges, MPH*

Substance use and abuse often coexist with anger, aggression, and violence. Anger and violent behaviors have been shown to be both a cause for the initiation of drug and alcohol use and a consequence associated with using. Data from the Substance Abuse and Mental Health Services Administration's National Household Survey on Drug Abuse found that 40 percent of frequent drug users reported engaging in some form of aggressive or violent behavior (SAMHSA 2002). Individuals who abuse drugs or alcohol are more likely to have an external locus of control, higher levels of anxiety, and markedly higher levels of aggression. Addicts and alcoholics are also less likely to have control over angry impulses. Addicted individuals have also been found to experience, express, and control anger differently than a matched control group of non-drug users. Drug abusers have higher state and trait levels of anger, higher angry temperaments, greater anger reactions, greater outward displays of anger, and lower control of their anger than controls without addictions (De Moja and Spielberger 1997). This suggests that those afflicted with addiction have a harder time controlling their anger and expressing it appropriately.

Alcoholics are also more likely to become frustrated and angry compared to those who don't have problems with alcohol. One reason for this is that alcohol may give an alcoholic the courage to act on feelings of anger due to decreased inhibitions. It has been found that alcohol weakens the brain mechanisms that typically control impulsive behaviors (Gaskell 2010). Further, the inability to manage anger often stems from excessive alcohol use, thus promoting a negative feedback loop for anger, aggression, and the abuse of alcohol, a rather dangerous cycle of anger. Alcohol also damages the parts of the brain responsible for controlling emotions, making it more difficult to keep anger in check. Alcohol can also breed anger because family, work, financial, and health problems are often experienced when using alcohol (Pearson 2010).

When examining the brain scans of individuals with aggressive problems, impairments were found in the prefrontal brain areas involved in decision making, brain regions in the amygdala that process negative inputs, and regions in the angular gyrus involved in calculating risks. These brain areas involved in moral judgments help show the chemical and neural responses of anger. When we get angry, not only do heart rate and artery tension rise, but testosterone production increases, stress levels decrease in the brain, and the left frontal lobe becomes more active. When we are angry, we don't dwell on negativity but instead are more focused on taking action (experienced through acts of aggression), and this focus triggers activity in the left hemisphere (Brogaard 2010). Interestingly, these same processes are also implicated in a reward mechanism, which makes anger that much more difficult to control. In a study of anger rewards, researchers found that high-testosterone people learned a complicated sequence quicker when an angry face followed the sequence than when a neutral or happy face followed it. Low-testosterone people did not learn any faster regardless of the emotional expression on the face that followed. The difference was even greater when the faces were shown at a level below conscious awareness, suggesting that the anger input to the brain promotes a reflexive response that is difficult to control. Since triggering anger in others is one way to dominate them, this can feel like a reward to high-testosterone people, because high testosterone is associated with a desire to dominate. Anger is thus rewarding for some people, making it further difficult to regulate (Brogaard 2010). When these findings are coupled with the presence of addiction, these effects are further exacerbated.

Understanding anger is critically important to its management. Anger is a natural emotion experienced in a fight-or-flight situation resulting from our feeling threatened in some way. The threat can be either real or perceived, as both are just as powerful to our brains. Anger is a force we project to push away or combat our individualized threat. Common triggers of anger are stress, significant relationships, family, driving, work, or anger in others (e.g., bullies). Physiologically, anger stems from the fear and anxiety elicited from dangerous or threatening situations (again, this can be real or perceived). First, we perceive a threat. While the perceived threat is still playing out, anxiety ensues because we want that threat to go away. If the anxiety goes unnoticed either by others or ourselves, then relief from the discomfort of anxiety is not provided. As such, feelings of frustration and anger can result to combat the threat. Anger responses can also be a reaction to emotional pain, wherein the mind perceives emotional pain, maltreatment, or abuse (e.g., feeling disrespected, undervalued, unappreciated, unrecognized, or powerless to have any sort of change or input). Anger can also result from misplaced blame. Anger could thus either be directed at others in an attempt to "get even" or to punish someone for the elicited feeling or directed at the self in a form of self-harm resulting from self-judgments based on using others as a comparison (e.g., feelings of rejection, isolation, or abandonment). Researchers have emphasized the need to distinguish between the experience and expression of anger in this way. When anger is experienced, it may be suppressed or directed inward, expressed toward other persons or objects in the environment, or controlled by preventing its expression ("keeping the lid on"). The outward expression of anger may involve the manifestation of aggressive behaviors such as verbal criticism, insults, use of profanity, assault of others, or destruction of objects in the environment (Spielberger et al. 1988). Individual anger expression styles thus vary, therefore emphasizing the need to individually tailor and explore root causes of anger and reaction tendencies in treatment.

Potter-Efron and Potter-Efron's book *Letting Go of Anger* delineates three broad groupings of anger: masked, chronic, and explosive. People who mask their anger do not let others see it because they believe anger is essentially useless, scary, and harmful. These individuals are highly uncomfortable with their anger and avoid being angry at all costs because anger in them elicits feelings of shame. This shame can be further exacerbated by the shame accompanying addictive behaviors. Anger is thus "stuffed" rather than expressed and internalized across all situations, even when expressing it would be appropriate. In the event that anger is expressed, it is done in a passive-aggressive way to get back at the target by "forgetting" to do something, wherein the angry person can avoid responsibility and also project a consequence to the anger source. Individuals of this anger style consequently often have a difficult time setting boundaries and limits by saying no or being assertive, which can promulgate existing difficulties in this arena as related to recovery (1995).

Individuals with chronic anger exemplify a persistent pattern of anger constantly, wherein anger dominates their lives. Often, chronically angry individuals develop resentments to people or institutions that they believe have harmed them. This is frequently associated with overinterpreting maltreatment and projecting excessively angry responses than a situation would otherwise warrant. Chronic anger can also have a moralistic flavor to it that may be paired with splitting: "I am right, others are wrong"; "I am good and others are evil personified." The combination of chronic anger and splitting is that commonly seen in individuals with borderline personality disorder. Not surprisingly, individuals with chronic anger are frequently unhappy and have a nihilistic disposition. Attitudes found within this anger style include, "life sucks and then you die," "people can't be trusted," "love predicts betrayal and abandonment," "hopes and dreams are frustrating illusions," and "bad always follows good but good never follows bad." Feelings of sadness may trail behind chronic anger, thus reinforcing the chronically angry individual's life perception and discouraging change (Potter-Efron and Potter-Efron 1995).

The third typology delineated by Potter-Efron and Potter-Efron is explosive anger. This anger style is characterized by periodically losing control of anger and then getting irate. Anger in this style comes on very suddenly, quickly takes over, and leads individuals to do or say things they later regret. Anger exploders are highly confrontational. Sometimes, this anger is based in shame and results in "shame-rage." Other times, explosive anger is a sign of a deeper psychological hostility. Many with this style are rewarded by their behavior because it gets them what they want through intimidation and manipulation; yelling at an employee may have the effect of getting the employee to perform a specific task or carry out a certain activity to avoid getting yelled at again. Unfortunately, while this style of anger expression may obtain desired results specific to a situation, anger explosion also serves to make others afraid and withdrawn from the exploder and damages relationships in the long term. Finally, some anger exploders report "getting high" off being angry, feeling more alive, intense, and powerful through its expression. These "rageaholics" have become psychologically addicted to their anger. Anger creates a rush of adrenaline and other physiological responses that can be addicting and may create a sense of being "truly alive." Like other addictions, there is a tolerance build-up that ultimately requires bigger and bigger fights to satisfy the need and eventually results in harmful consequences to both others and the self (1995).

Recognizing and increasing awareness of one's individual anger style is crucial in its management. Given the high correlation between anger and addiction, treatment and management of anger is often addressed simultaneously in addictions treatment, usually through group therapy. Strategies for combating anger may vary both by situation and the individual, so learning and honing m ultiple methods for managing anger will provide both a diverse and extensive repertoire from which to pull in anger-eliciting situations and provide opportunities for preventing unhealthy expressions of anger. The following anger combating strategies may serve as a helpful starting point:

- Take a time out

    - Formally express your need for space in an angry situation and take the time to calm down, go for a walk, or obtain clarity before returning to the situation and addressing it assertively and rationally.

- Buy yourself some time

    - In certain situations, delaying a response until a later time may prevent a rash expression of anger or aggression and can allow for enhanced ability to make a sound decision.

- Practice relaxation

    - Taking the time to relax by unwinding in a nonstressful activity can calm the body and ease the mind, both of which will help curb unhealthy anger expression.

- Meditate

    - Not only is meditation good for enhancing mindfulness and holistic insight, but regular meditation actually helps prevent aggression by increasing awareness and providing focus. The practice of regular meditation for at least fifteen minutes a day has been associated not only with better outcomes for substance abuse, but also with decreased aggression and hostility.

- Seek to enhance your awareness and understanding of the situation

    - Trying to see the situation from the other person's point of view may help you determine a response that will be more effective and that they will be more receptive to hearing. Asking questions of the other person to clarify their understanding of the situation may be a good preemptive way of straightening out potential misunderstandings and miscommunications before making rash accusations.

- Increase positive thoughts of others

    - This strategy is particularly helpful in significant relationships with family or romantic partners. When faced with a situation that provokes an anger response, attempting to re-

**Positive Sobriety**

member or remind yourself of a positive quality or memorable experience with that individual can help curb your anger and prevent a potentially hurtful response.

- Work on assertiveness skills

    o Assertiveness training helps individuals with masked or hidden anger in particular by helping them to admit they have angry feelings just like everyone else. Assertiveness training teaches that you can overtly stand up for yourself and express yourself by stating clear boundaries and setting limits. It also helps increase positive communication to promote coming to a resolution.

- Visualize

    o Visualizing means crafting a new vision of the future and imagining yourself being angry when appropriate and using your anger well. Role-playing appropriate handling of anger helps solidify the new pattern of behavior in the brain and also increases the likelihood of using it.

- Identify the root cause of anger

    o Figuring out what is really making you angry is just as critical as figuring out the determinants and triggers of addiction. Sometimes the root causes may be the same, but often they are not. Differentiating root causes can help you to recognize the physical signs of anger and also allows you to make a commitment to change through calmness, moderation, and enhanced choices.

- Find an alternative activity to get the anger out

    o Aerobic physical activity and yoga have been shown effective in calming anger and also preventing its onset. This works by regulating emotions through the hormones released through physical activity and also lets the anger be expressed in a healthier modality.

- Think of the *Cow in the Parking Lot*

    o Scheff and Edmiston's 2010 book illustrates how anger can easily turn into amusement by changing your perspective: "Imagine you are circling a crowded parking lot when, just as you spot a space, another driver races ahead and takes it. Easy to imagine the rage. But now imagine that instead of another driver, a cow has lumbered into that parking space and settled down. The anger dissolves into bemusement. What really changed? You—your perspective." Simply changing one variable in a situation (a cow instead of another car) can transform a situation from one of anger to one of laughter. Picturing a docile cow instead of the person or situation that makes you angry not only makes for a funny visualization, but it also brings perspective back to the situation. Laughter may in fact be the best medicine.

# Post-Acute Withdrawal Syndrome (PAWS)

*Ethan Bickelhaupt, MD*

Post-acute withdrawal syndrome (PAWS) is a group of addictive disease symptoms and signs that occur as a result of abstinence from alcohol or other drugs, generally appearing seven to fourteen days after cessation and peaking between three and six months during abstinence, affecting each person differently. Originally termed "protracted alcohol withdrawal delirium," PAWS can occur intermittently or consistently or operate in a regenerative or degenerative pattern. It is a biopsychosocial syndrome resulting from the combination of damage to the nervous system caused by the drug and the psychological stress of coping without the substance. As mentioned in chapter 2, brain imaging has shown that for weeks and even months after use, there is decreased blood flow and activity in the areas of the brain necessary for feeling good and making good decisions. This damage is usually reversible with proper treatment, including adherence to a recovery program and complete abstinence. PAWS is typically identified as the inability to solve simple problems, often leading to diminished self-esteem, embarrassment, and fear of failure that interfere with a recovering person's life. Knowing that PAWS is a process and not having excessive expectations are very important in managing and overcoming the syndrome.

PAWS symptoms and signs include:

1) Inability to think clearly, including short attention span, impairment of abstract reasoning, and rigid and repetitive thinking. These factors are part of the executive function of the human brain.

2) Memory problems, including impaired short-term memory as well as difficulty remembering the past while under great stress and difficulty learning and retaining new information and developing related skills.

3) Emotional over- or under reaction, meaning inappropriate emotional responses to situations, whether heightened or deadened emotional responses, mostly due to a diminished capacity to cope with stress.

4) Sleep disturbances, either trouble sleeping or experiencing disturbing dreams, both of which tend to abate over time.

5) Physical coordination problems. These are uncommon but exhibited by dizziness, clumsiness, and being accident-prone.

6) Sensitivity to stress—again, inappropriate emotional responses to situations that normally would not warrant an extreme reaction. Heightened stress impacts the severity of each of the other symptoms and signs of PAWS.

Managing PAWS requires engaging in self-care activities such as relaxation, a healthy diet, exercising, incorporating spirituality, and living a balanced life (Miller 1994). This process generates a greater potential for happiness and the development of a level of serenity that permits a reduction in self-loathing and shame and makes greater hope possible.

In addition to enlisting professional help, talking to others who can be trusted not to criticize or minimize a person's current experiences can help with viewing the existing situation and behaviors more realistically, enhancing a social support network, and assisting in developing goals and solutions to problems in living. It is equally important to conduct self-examination, revisiting what may have contributed to PAWS symptoms and signs. This allows for mapping a new plan for the future.

# Relapse

*Wally Cross, RPH, MHS, CADC*

Relapse is a progressive process of a once-stable recovery system becoming so dysfunctional that returning to substance use is an option. There are several factors that can increase the potential for relapse. These are long history of relapsing, long chemical use history, comorbid psychiatric diagnoses, low level of disease acceptance, low self-efficacy, poor investment in AA, weak support system, and low level of stability.

Just as breaking a pervasive use pattern is very difficult, breaking the habit of relapsing is equally so. Often, once a person has relapsed, the option for doing so again is more viable. It may happen sooner and with less inner dispute. Thought patterns about substances and use of substances become hardwired in the brain over time, and in order for sobriety to remain intact, often the thoughts associated with use need to be changed. Instead of thinking that relapse might be an option, one needs to think that it is never an option. AA addresses rewiring and retraining the brain to think about substances in a different way by employing repetition and using particular language specific to the AA commitment to recovery to talk about substances and substance use. The repetitive language helps solidify the idea in your mind so it becomes reflective of your new life.

People with a long history of substance use generally have a higher potential for relapsing. Recent studies show that something called "cortical thinning" occurs as a result of continued abuse of alcohol and increases the risk of relapse (K. Rando et al. 2011). In fact, recent studies at Yale (Sinha 2011) used MRI studies showing that decrease in gray matter (what constitutes the frontal areas of the brain) correlated with increased relapse. There may come a time when these scans can be more affordable and available and help us know who is at greater risk for relapse.

Those who have been in addiction for three years are more likely to succeed without relapse than those whose addiction has been going on for twelve years. However, sometimes a longer addiction provides a heightened motivation for change. Those who have spent a longer time in addiction may feel "done" with their addiction in a way that someone with less time in addiction may not feel.

It is common for people that come to treatment for addictions to have symptoms of or a full diagnosis of a psychiatric condition including depression, bipolar disorder, anxiety, eating disorders, chronic pain, cognitive impairment, or personality disorders. These diagnoses and the corresponding symptoms impact treatment in a variety of ways. For example, people experiencing the manic phase of bipolar disorder lose the ability to make good choices, as their capacity for judgment is severely impaired. This may contribute to someone deciding to use during a manic phase when they may not make that choice under other circumstances. For this reason, addressing and controlling symptomatic and unstable psychiatric issues is very important to avoiding relapse.

Some people erroneously believe that if they originally had a problem with narcotics that got them into treatment but never abused alcohol, once they leave treatment, they can use alcohol within normal limits. However, addiction transcends all substances. People who think they are not as bad off as others they see in treatment or recovery may feel like they can get away with not investing as much of themselves into aspects of recovery such as going to meetings, obtaining a sponsor and maintaining contact, or adhering to abstinence, which increases the probability that they will relapse. Addiction is a chronic disease, and until the addict accepts this and the implications of a continued effort throughout life to maintain healthy sobriety, risk of relapse goes up.

Having a strong support system is necessary for recovery. Sometimes personal feelings of shame overwhelm the addicted person to the point where they hide aspects of treatment from their family, mostly the importance of participating in a recovery system. The family system goes through a change when the addict decides to pursue recovery, and many issues can arise from this. Sometimes families are not supportive either, due to lack of education or feelings of anger. These things can be examined in a family program within a treatment program or in family therapy. Other family dynamics are discussed in "Family Program" in chapter 3.

# AA: 1 and 2

*Wally Cross, RPH, MHS, CADC*

Finding an AA program that fits you is vital to success in maintaining abstinence. There are a plethora of meetings that address different populations, such as men only, women only, atheists or agnostics, smokers, nonsmokers, and others. When deciding on a group, your sponsor may be able to help. You can attend your sponsor's group or go to one on your own. For your main group, you should look for certain qualities, including that the members have similar backgrounds to yours; that the group is comprised of at least some members who have a good, healthy recovery who can serve as models; that group members who enjoy being together and doing things outside of the group; and that meetings discuss different topics each week. Generally, you should try to find a group that has from ten to thirty members. Depending on your style of communicating, you may feel more comfortable in a smaller group than in a larger group. It is important to participate in the groups to help you feel connected, as feeling more connected will decrease the likelihood that you will drop out. When choosing a sponsor, you should look for someone who you trust, who is the same gender, who has at least two years of recovery, who has time to spend with you, whom you feel comfortable with, and who will be directive and teach you the steps and be honest about your progress. You should shop around for both a sponsor and a group. If you give the group and sponsor an honest try and find that it is not the type of relationship that works for you in cultivating your recovery, you can always find another. Sticking to these suggestions and making the effort will effectively increase your odds of staying sober.

# Shame and Guilt

*Barb Laukaitis, CADC*

Shame is a part of all people's emotional experience. In its healthy form, it outlines one's limits, exhibited in feeling moderate shyness in unfamiliar situations, slight embarrassment for making a mistake, and an ability to feel vulnerable and humble enough to ask for help when it's needed. In its toxic form, shame is internalized and becomes a strong motivator for self-destructive behavior and a great impediment to healthy growth and development. Shame differs from guilt in that guilt says, "I made a mistake and there is a way to recover," and shame says, "I am a mistake and there is no relief" (Bradshaw 2005). Guilt is thinking that I made a mistake, whereas shame is thinking that others think you made a mistake, whether you did or not. Because we cannot control what others think, we cannot forgive or relieve shame, leading to repression. Moderation of shame requires mindfulness to let go of judging and blaming oneself and others—thereby transcending the low self-esteem that comes from being dependent on others' judgment of ourselves.

Addicts and people with other compulsive behaviors suffer from internalized shame more than others. Shame initially becomes internalized when one's parents (primary caregivers) are shame based but acting shamelessly, meaning they express their own internalized shame by projecting it onto the child and being overly critical; expecting perfection; abusing children physically, sexually, or emotionally; or otherwise exhibiting controlling behavior. Through these behaviors, the parent is able to cover their own shame by acting powerful. It is during childhood when we are the most needy and also when we are vulnerable to being hurt the most. The aforementioned behaviors perpetuated by the primary caregivers result in the child being emotionally abandoned, which precipitates an undercurrent of mistrust of others, as the child and eventually the adult expects abandonment from all relationships. After all, if one's parents don't love the child, how can anyone else? Children idealize their parents, so when this dynamic is present in the family, the child believes it is something wrong with them that makes their parents act in such ways, internalizes that shame, and grows into a shame-based adult who is susceptible to repeating the same patterns in their relationships with other adults and their own children.

Abandonment leads to a loss of the authentic self, or an inability to be who one truly is, due to internalized feelings of personal inadequacy and worthlessness and thoughts that one is defective from the imposition of shame. The shame becomes internal and contemptuous, leading the person to dissociate from themselves. They become superhuman (perfectionist, overly ambitious, or indignant) or subhuman (sloppy, reclusive, criminal). Addiction seeps in and fills the hole of shame; the person relies on external experiences for happiness, as they are unable to generate happiness within themselves. Shame and addiction operate in a cycle such that the shame creates distorted thinking ("I'm worthless; I'm defective") that leads to acting out (engaging in the addiction) that becomes life-damaging ("I lost my job; I contracted AIDS from sharing drug needles"), further proving the underlying message, "I am flawed because I did this to myself."

Fixing the shame is a crucial step in fixing the pattern of addiction. If the shame is left unresolved, it will continue to motivate self-destructive behaviors and manifest in another way—binge eating, compulsive gambling, or any number of compulsive behaviors. Bradshaw (2005) discusses confronting shame through surrendering, socializing with others through therapy or a twelve-step group, surfacing the buried memories related to the onset of shame and disclosing them, being sensitive to the system of shame and enhancing awareness of one's own shame-based behaviors, loving oneself enough to forgive oneself for maladaptive behaviors, and gaining an inner life and spirituality. Embracing shame puts one in touch with oneself, especially the inner child who was hurt, and allows for the self to be integrated. The collaborative and reciprocal environment inherent in AA is very helpful for confronting shame. The well-known slogans of AA such as "one day at a time," "this too shall pass," and others provide people with language to reassure themselves as they go through the process of recovery. As important as it is to promoting the overall health of the recovering addict, fixing shame does not mean you can then drink successfully—shame may be the main underlying psychological process contributing to the addiction, but it doesn't encompass the whole of the disease.

The second part of this lecture involves having patients think of and then share a memory of being shamed, preferably before the age of twelve. Then, they sit in a circle, close their eyes, and think of a message they would have liked to have received in contrast to the shame they felt. Each person then gets up, goes around the room, and whispers that message to all other people in the circle. Through this exercise, each member of the group has received a number of positive messages, an experience that is often very different from the barrage of negative messages they have received throughout life and tend to repeat to themselves. The group as a whole processes the experience by discussing whether it was easier to give or to receive the messages, what felt uncomfortable, and which of the messages they may have identified with most. The purpose of the group exercise is to realize that the hurt has been done and that the perpetrators of the hurt will not fix it, and instead the responsibility now lies within each person to heal themselves and effectively break the cycle so as not to pass those same messages on to further generations. Addressing the shame is congruent with the idea of promoting positive sobriety by focusing on the inner self, cultivating an inner life, and learning how to generate happiness from within.

# Codependency

*Robert Smith, LSW, CADC*

The importance of relationships between human beings supersedes all other aspects of what makes us who we are and how we operate in the world. Plain and simple, human beings are not meant to live an insular, reclusive life void of contact with other humans, as it is maladaptive and in opposition to the tenets of healthy attachment theory. An explanation of attachment theory is necessary, as it provides the foundation for further discussion of the topic of codependency and healthy interdependence.

Within attachment theory, *attachment* means an affectional bond or tie between an individual and an attachment figure; it describes the dynamics of long-term relationships between humans. These dynamics of relationship patterns and behaviors are usually established in early childhood and carried into adulthood. Hopefully, individuals grow up in an environment of healthy, open-system families where relationship patterns and behaviors are accepting, adaptive, malleable, and flexible. However this is not always realistic, especially in a family system where alcohol and drugs exist at the epicenter of the relationship dynamics, thus establishing a closed system where controlling, manipulating, and fixing behaviors become the norm.

Codependency stems from a dysfunctional pattern of relating developed early in childhood in response to stressful family dynamics. These stressful family dynamics include addiction, abuse, mental illness, physical illness, divorce, neglect, or many others that characteristically contain an emotionally abusive or unavailable parent or parents. The result of a closed-system family that is dysfunctional, either through mental illness or alcohol or drug use, can be devastating to individuals in the system resulting in inappropriate alliances, triangulation, and possible enmeshment between individuals who are incapable of self-differentiation. Hence, the perfect storm of unhealthy codependency is created and firmly established within the schema of individuals. As with most cognitions and behaviors, the degree of codependency individuals exhibit has much variance along a spectrum.

Since the inception of the word *codependency*, the term has be misinterpreted and used in an incorrect way to the point that any form of codependency is viewed as pathological. Codependency exists on spectrum, and there is a healthy form of existing in relationships, which is better known as "interdependency." Interdependency can be viewed as being whole and balanced persons who are able to share with and join in the healthy resources of relationships with others deemed important to their lives. Interdependency facilitates an even greater expansion in experiencing life than independency and certainly more than codependency, as individuals now have unlimited access to even more love, success, and happiness than they could have provided for themselves. Unfortunately, entrenched patterns of dysfunctional relational dynamics as well as alcohol and drug use set the stage for individuals to become codependent, preventing movement to independence and then finally to interdependence.

Codependency is a dysfunctional relationship with the self characterized by living through or for another, attempting to control others, blaming others, feeling a sense of victimization, attempting to "fix" others, and experiencing intense anxiety around intimacy. Individuals do not have to have an official diagnosis of codependency to exhibit these maladaptive behaviors and cognitions that are compulsive and repetitive and carried from one relationship to another. Having features and traits of codependency is enough to affect individuals' interpersonal relationships in such an unhealthy way that harmful emotional and physical consequences affect the well-being of all individuals involved in the relationships.

Physical problems often result from untreated codependency. These may include gastrointestinal disturbances such as colitis or ulcers, migraine headaches, nonspecific rashes and skin problems, high blood pressure, insomnia and other sleep disorders, and other stress-related physical illnesses. In addition, emotional problems such as depression, anxiety, relationship dysfunctions, and cycling between hyperactivity and lethargy are evident in many codependents.

## Common Symptoms of Codependency

| Lack of self-confidence in making decisions, no sense of power in making choices | Feelings of fear, insecurity, inadequacy, guilt, hurt, and shame, which are denied |
|---|---|
| Isolation and fear of people, resentment of authority figures | Fear of expressing anger or bottling anger up till it explodes |
| Low self-esteem, which is often projected onto others (e.g., "Why don't *they* get their act together?") | Difficulty developing or sustaining meaningful relationships |
| Belief that others cause or are responsible for the codependent's emotions. | Constantly seeking approval and affirmation, yet having a compromised sense of self |

**Positive Sobriety**

| Judging oneself or others without mercy. | Hypersensitivity to criticism |
|---|---|
| Being either super-responsible or super-irresponsible (or alternating between these) | Inability to see alternatives to situations, thus responding very impulsively |
| Overreacting to change (or intense fear of or inability to deal with change) | |

If individuals have difficulty determining whether codependency exists in their lives, the following list of useful questions will assist them in identification.

- Do you feel responsible for other people—their feelings, thoughts, actions, choices, wants, needs, well-being, and destiny?

- Do you feel compelled to help people solve their problems or try to take care of their feelings?

- Do you find it easier to feel and express anger about injustices done to others than about injustices done to you?

- Do you feel safest and most comfortable when you are giving to others?

- Do you feel insecure and guilty when someone gives to you?

- Do you feel empty, bored, or worthless if you don't have someone else to take care of, a problem to solve, or a crisis to deal with?

- Are you often unable to stop talking, thinking, or worrying about other people and their problems?

- Do you lose interest in your own life when you are in love?

- Do you stay in relationships that don't work and tolerate abuse in order to keep people loving you?

- Do you leave bad relationships only to form new ones that don't work either?

The repetitive characteristics of codependency are like many other behaviors and cognitions individuals act out unconsciously in that in codependency, individuals lack insight and are unaware of the dysfunction and harm inflicted to the self. It is paramount for individuals who identify as codependents or who are living with codependency to work toward the healthy goal of changing already established relationships or moving into relationships or relational patterns that are interdependent. Hence, through different therapy modalities and self-help groups such as Codependents Anonymous, individuals can move along the spectrum from codependence to independence to interdependence in their attachments and relationships with other human beings.

# Impact of Addiction on Loved Ones

*Kathy Bettinardi-Angres APN, MS, RN, CADC*

The patients are only minimally aware of the impact of their disease on their loved ones. The reasons include their own need to focus on self for survival and the immense shame that many feel regarding this topic. It is, however, important that they have a sense of what their family members are experiencing in order to improve communication and heighten empathy.

The family members actually pass through their own stages of early recovery immediately after the patient is admitted to rehab. These stages are easily identified with the acronym DRAFT:

D: Despair. The initial sensation felt by loved ones when the reality of the need for medical and psychological intervention is necessary for the survival of the patient.

R: Relief. The welcome feeling that is expressed when the patient leaves home and is initially sober because the tension in the home is reduced and the possibility of hope is restored.

A: Anger. All family members and loved ones experience anger, but they each express it differently. Some may be directly angry at the patient, others displace the anger toward a workplace, for example, and still others may repress their anger and exhibit physical ailments.

F: Fear. Fear is always about future relapse and the consequences of the patient's use that impact family and loved ones.

T: Tolerance. Not to be confused with acceptance, tolerance happens when the family members start to incorporate the reality of recovery but still find it difficult to avoid feeling somewhat special or different from the "hard core" addicts and alcoholics.

Family members may experience the pain of loving someone with addiction similar to loving one who experiences a trauma. This is not to say it is the same, but according to the DSM IV-R, the symptoms of posttraumatic stress disorder are alarmingly similar to those feelings experienced by family members of addicts and alcoholics. PTSD is "a common anxiety disorder that develops after exposure to a single or series of traumatic events. This trauma can be defined as a threat to the physical integrity of self or others.

Interestingly, the family and loved ones of addicts and alcoholics often identify with this disorder and feel a sense of relief that they are "not crazy." This is not an attempt to diagnose significant others, only a way to validate their suffering and move them to begin their own recovery.

Patients and loved ones alike need to pursue their own individual recovery in order to heal the family as a whole and allow for future growth and deeper connection among all family members. The accepted treatments for PTSD include psychotherapy, EMDR, and yoga. These therapies have also been effective in treating loved ones of addicts and alcoholics.

# Stages of Change

*Robert Smith, LSW, CADC*

Change in a broad context is inevitable and constant in the life of each individual; sometimes change is done consciously and by choice, and other times change is not done by choice but rather is beyond the individual's control. For individuals with addictive disease who use harmful substances, change to cease use of the substances is paramount for physical, mental, emotional, and spiritual well-being. Originally created in the late 1970s and early 1980s by theoreticians Prochaska and DiClemente, the Stages of Change model was used as an intervention to get individuals to stop smoking even if they did not want to stop or were ambivalent about stopping.

Under the guise of the scientific name the Transtheoretical Model (TTM), the Stages of Change as a substance abuse treatment intervention is one of the most successful evidence-based practice techniques to move individuals from active addiction to abstinence and sustained recovery. In the realm of addiction, the Stages of Change model assesses an individual's readiness to employ new coping skills and healthier behaviors and provides strategies or processes of conscious change that direct the individual through each stage to achieve sustained, long-term abstinence.

Although the main focus of the Stages of Change model is on the stage the individual is in with regard to the use of, abuse of, or dependency on drugs and alcohol, it is imperative the individual understand he or she can apply these stages to all areas of life. A holistic application of the Stages of Change model reinforces and supports the holistic approach to recovery, in which an individual is conscious about the importance of having internal balance and being in balance with the external environment. Because such areas as interpersonal relationships, vocation, and general health behaviors have a direct impact on an individual's recovery, emphasis is placed on the individual having the introspection of which stage in a particular area of his or her life is and of the processes by which he or she can move to the next healthier adaptive stage.

The Stages of Change model consists of five distinct and identifiable stages that are most useful in treating addiction but are universal to all aspects of an individual's life. It is important to note these stages are not linear but cyclical, as an individual may move from one stage to the next and then back to the previous stage. Ideally, healthy movement through the Stages of Change is upward, although lessons are learned in regression to an early stage. The following have been identified as the Stages of Change model:

**Stage 1: Precontemplation (Not Ready)**

Individuals at this stage do not intend to start the healthy behavior, in this case, the cessation of drugs or alcohol. They may be unaware of the need to change and are likely to use immature defense mechanisms such as denial. These individuals will vehemently deny they have a problem with drugs or alcohol even if they have experienced a major negative consequence as a result of use. At this stage, individuals are educated and encouraged to weigh the benefits and burdens, the pros and cons of their substance use. Precontemplators typically underestimate the pros of changing and overestimate the cons—they lack self-awareness.

**Stage 2: Contemplation (Getting Ready)**

At this stage, individuals intend to start the healthy behavior of quitting drugs or alcohol in the future. Whether through a series of negative consequences or self-awareness, individuals have accepted at some level that an alcohol- or drug-using problem exists. Thus, the scale of pros and cons has tipped, and the cons of continued use outweigh the pros. At this stage, usually a varied leverage exists in the individual's life pushing for behavior change. Individuals may remain in this stage for an extended period, their self-awareness riddled futile and turned to ambivalence by the continued use of maladaptive defense mechanisms. An individual's ambivalence is at its strongest point regarding continuing to use alcohol or drugs.

**Stage 3: Preparation (Ready)**

Individuals at this stage are ready to start taking action in the very near future. They do the research and take realistic steps that they believe can help them make the healthy behavior a part of their lives. For instance, individuals may inform friends and family that they want to change their behavior or research substance abuse treatment facilities for an appropriate fit.

**Stage 4: Action**

Individuals with addictive disease who have reached this stage of change have stopped using substances. A catalyst or a new act that is tangible has become part of the individual's life, such as admitting into a substance abuse treatment facility, going to twelve-step meetings, or seeing a therapist for psychotherapy. In a timeline, this stage can be defined as abstinence within the last six months. Because of the newness of the change, individuals are highly charged and fragile at this point; thus, a reward system for the behavior change is imperative to prevent the individual from returning to using substances. Individuals in this stage are taught life skills for the ongoing commitment to abstinence such as substituting activities related to the unhealthy behavior with healthy activities and avoiding situations that prompt them to behave in unhealthy ways.

**Stage 5: Maintenance**

After achieving more than six months of abstinence, individuals enter the stage of maintenance. Maintenance continues for an indefinite period of time and involves being able to successfully avoid temptations that would result in using substances again. The individual has gained a self-awareness that abstinence is constantly the goal and is personally worthwhile and meaningful. Thoughts of using substances may occasionally occur, but healthy coping strategies and practiced life skills protect the individual from relapsing and returning to a lifestyle of using.

While relapse is not favorable, it is realistic in individuals with addictive disease, so it must be addressed as the elephant in the room. Relapse is not a stage of the Stages of Change model; rather, it is an event when an individual has returned to using substances, usually for a short time. Many individuals who successfully stop using substances do not follow a straight path to a lifetime of abstinence. Rather, they may cycle through the Stages several times.

For the Stages of Change model to be successful in cessation of drugs or alcohol and other unhealthy behaviors or lifestyles, the following must occur when individuals move from being precomtemplators to maintainers.

1) The presence of a decisional balance exists in which the individuals are increasingly aware that the advantages (the pros) of changing outweigh the disadvantages (the cons).

2) An existence of self-efficacy is present. Individuals have confidence they can make and maintain changes in situations that tempt them to return to their unhealthy behavior, using alcohol and drugs.

3) Strategies and coping skills known as "processes of change," which help make and maintain change, are practiced. The ten processes are:

- Consciousness-raising: "I recall information people gave me on how to stop using alcohol or drugs."

- Dramatic relief: "I react emotionally to warnings about using alcohol or drugs."

- Self-reevaluation: "My dependency on alcohol or drugs makes me feel disappointed in myself."

- Environmental reevaluation: "I consider the view that drinking and using drugs can be harmful to my external world."

- Social liberation: "I realize that society is more supportive of my healthy behavior of stopping the use alcohol or drugs."

- Stimulus control: "I remove things from my home that remind me of drinking and using drugs."

- Helping relationship: "I have someone who listens when I need to talk about my alcohol or drug use."

- Counterconditioning: "I find that doing other things with my Friday and Saturday nights is a good substitute for going out drinking at the bars."

- Reinforcement management: "I reward myself when I don't drink alcohol and use drugs."

- Self-liberation: "I make commitments not to drink alcohol or use drugs."

# Trauma and Recovery

*Jeffrey W. Zacharias LCSW, CADC*

According to the American Psychiatric Association DSM-IV, trauma is "the exposure to an extreme stressor involving direct personal experience of an event that involves actual or threatened death or serious injury, or threat to one's physical integrity; or witnessing an event that involves death, injury or a threat to the physical integrity of another person; or learning about unexpected or violent death, serious harm, or threat of death or injury experienced by a family member of close associate." In other words, an event that causes an unusually high level of emotional stress affecting an individual on a long term basis can be described as traumatic. Trauma is a subjective experience based on the emotion evoked by the experience rather than the actual experience itself. Therefore, there can be as many definitions of trauma as there are individuals. Unable to deal effectively with trauma, individuals may employ maladaptive coping skills such as the use of drugs and alcohol to cope with their pain leading to the potential development of an addiction. The correlation between trauma and addiction is complex and there is a critical need to address both trauma and addiction concurrently so an individual can heal their mind, body and soul.

Trauma can have a devastating impact on an individual and their worldview. Feeling a sense of heightened danger, an individual may develop a belief system that the world is not a safe place which is a common reaction to trauma. An individual begins to doubt they can take care of themselves or those around them in meaningful ways. As a result, comorbid diagnoses such as depression, anxiety and/or panic disorder as well as dissociation may occur. Additionally, flashbacks, under- or over-reactions to daily life events, increased feelings of anger/rage/hopelessness/worthlessness and isolation due to a heightened sense of danger are common responses to trauma. Post-Traumatic Stress Disorder (PTSD) is the most common form of comorbid diagnoses. Interestingly enough, studies have shown that 70 percent of people have experienced at least one traumatic event in their lifetime with 8 percent of the population having an increase in the intensity of the event rather than abatement in their symptoms. It has also been estimated that 40 percent of individuals, particularly women, who present for inpatient substance abuse treatment also meet the criteria for PTSD. Women have increasingly been shown to suffer from PTSD due to domestic violence in their lives. PTSD becomes quite complicated to treat especially if there is addiction issues involved. A cycle develops in which an individual wants to temporarily relieve their PTDS symptoms through the use of drugs/alcohol but then when the individual begins to go through withdrawals from drugs/alcohol their original PTSD symptoms return and even be intensified.

Trauma can be broken down into two subsets – "small t" trauma and "Big T Trauma." Big T trauma, the more well-known type of trauma, involves a threat to physical safety be it sexual, mental, verbal or physical in nature. Examples of Big T trauma might include being involved in a car accident, domestic violence, being in natural disasters such as earthquakes or being involved in war. "Small t Trauma" may not routinely be viewed as traumatic as they are common life events that are upsetting on the surface but not thought of as traumatizing long term. Examples of small t trauma might include the death of a pet, divorce, being bullied in school or loss of a job. Due to the individualistic nature of trauma to each person, a Big T trauma can be as debilitating as a small t trauma and the emotional wounds can be equally as intense and disturbing. Both types of trauma influence a person's world view and unless with dealt with in a healthy manner – i.e. individual therapy, treatment - can be equally as devastating. Time alone isn't enough to heal trauma and left untreated can be seen in a very similar vein to that of addiction - progressive and fatal unless treated.

In his book "Waking the Tiger: Healing Trauma", Peter Levine writes "Trauma is like a straightjacket that binds the mind and body in frozen fear. Paradoxically, it is also a portal that can lead us to awakening and freedom." In other words, the key to healing is to take the fear and the energy associated with the trauma and use it for personal healing rather than remaining locked in the trauma. Recovery is more effective if an individual goes slowly and allows the healing to occur at their pace rather than enveloping the mind and body in fear once again. Much work has been done in recent years in how to heal from trauma while recovering from active addiction. There has been proven efficacy in several methods most notably Eye Movement Desensitization and Reprocessing (EMDR).

Eye Movement Desensitization and Reprocessing (EMDR) works by using rapid eye movement to activate the trauma, brings those memories to the forefront of the mind where they are able to be processed and then restructure the memory of the event into something much more manageable. EMDR is most often effective when used with other more traditional types of therapy. In the case of an individual who is dealing with both trauma and addiction, a combination of EMDR and traditional Cognitive Behavioral Therapy (CBT) may be the right combination of interventions to ameliorate these co-occurring issues. Studies that have been done up to this point have shown EMDR to be effective for dealing with the following traumas: loss/injury of a loved one, car/work accidents, physical/sexual abuse, being a victim and/or witness of a violent crime, childhood abuse/trauma, depression, anxiety, phobias and overwhelming fears.

Another form of therapy that can be helpful in dealing with the co-occurring issues of trauma and addiction is Dialectical Behavioral Therapy (DBT). DBT, a form of Cognitive Behavioral Therapy (CBT), has shown great success in recent years as it assists individuals in developing concrete skills to deal with overwhelming emotions that may have resulted from earlier trauma. Once able to process these emotions in a healthier way, the individual is less likely to turn to drugs and/or alcohol as a coping mechanism. An individual in DBT engages in four modules that focus on four groups of skills: core mindfulness, interpersonal effectiveness, emotional regulation and distress tolerance. The four primary modes of treatment that are offered in order to do this are: individual therapy, group therapy, telephone contact and therapist consultation.

Trauma, whether Big T or little t, is complex, individualistic and recovery from it is difficult. If survivors of trauma develop a drug and/or alcohol addiction as an adverse coping mechanism, the recovery process is further complicated and both issues can be progressive and fatal. Treatment for these issues should not be compartmentalized but rather dealt with concurrently in order for the individual to have the best outcome. With the right form of therapy and interventions, an individual can recover mind, body and soul from both trauma and addiction.

# 5. Who Are You? Personality and Addiction

Personality—we've all got one. And even if we fall into a particular category—let's say, a histrionic personality, in which we need to be the center of attention—we are all unique. Our personalities are so complex and personal they are like snowflakes or fingerprints. Our personalities are who we are, or who we think we are. But how fixed is this self we travel through life with?

## Self, No Self

The "self," that sense of "I," can be elusive and misleading. The composite of who we think we are is constantly changing. There are any numbers of competing priorities at any given moment that arise in our consciousness, yet there is a necessary sense of history, personality, and adaptive style that endures. This sense of self can be hardened and can perpetuate the myth that we are somehow unified and solid in our constantly shifting persona. Paradoxically, the more secure our sense of self is, the easier it is to really see the illusion of self and have success in transcending it. Addiction is notorious for producing disruption in self structures. Even in the case of someone who had a relatively secure self-development prior to addiction, the addictive process will invariably gnaw away at this secure self. The progression of any addiction involves increasing self-centeredness and a growing inability to delay gratification and tolerate frustration along with a deterioration of character development.

The Buddhist conception of "no self, or "anatman," challenges the Western emphasis on self in the pursuit of self-esteem. In David Galin's essay "The Concept 'Self' and 'Person' in Buddhism and in Western Psychology" describes the Buddhist "correct view" of the self (2001). Galin states, "The Self is not seen as an entity or as a substance, or as an essence but as a dynamic process, a shifting web of relations among evanescent aspects of the person such as perceptions, ideas, and desires." He further defines the self as "the organizations of subsystems" that can include self-regulating, self-monitoring, and self-awareness derivatives (Galin 2001). This more flexible, dynamic conception of self is critical to the development of a positive sobriety. Hayes captures the problems associated with a "fixed" sense of self in what he calls "Cognitive Fusion" (Hayes et al. 1999). In his Acceptance and Commitment Therapy, or ACT approach, Hayes refers to this fusion as the process wherein the person and the mind become fused. That is, people confuse their thoughts and feelings as facts rather as simply constructions of the mind that are transient by nature. The clinging to a rigid, unchanging sense of self, or a "me," is both inaccurate and can be nonadaptive (Hayes et al. 1999, 2004).

The emphasis here is on cultivating the capacity to *observe* thoughts and feelings rather than to *react* to them. This ultimately requires the development of a more flexible and fluid sense of self, whereby the "me" is more river than rock. Mindfulness-based cognitive behavioral therapy has demonstrated effectiveness in reducing relapse in depression, and the emphasis is on changing core beliefs and faulty, dangerous thinking patterns (Segal et al. 2001). This is best illustrated by slogans in twelve-step recovery circles such as "your best thinking got you here" and "when you are in your head, you are behind enemy lines," which are references to these thinking errors. In terms of folk wisdom, they can mean, "don't take yourself so seriously."

Dysfunctional thinking patterns typically lead to behavioral patterns that can be injurious to self and others. Cognitive reactivity, as described by Z. Segal and colleagues, refers to the downward spiral of thought when rumination dominates thinking (2001. Studies exploring the impact of cognition on relapse of depression suggest that patients in a relapse state are more vulnerable to the cognitions and motivations present during a previous relapse state.

Z. Segal and colleagues' mindfulness approach to cognitive therapy techniques shifts the emphasis to recognizing dysfunctional thinking and maladaptive core beliefs when they occur. However, instead of trying to change or restructure this belief system, the approach is to step back and observe the process. In this manner, the consequences of thoughts, to oneself and others, can be observed without self-judgment or criticism or the mandate to make immediate changes to cognitions. Instead, the thought processes can be observed, and simultaneously the observing ego functions can be enhanced. A fluid sense of self that is not fused with thought allows for change (Segal 2001).

# Narcissism, Addictive Personality, and Quantum Change

### Addictive Personality?

An interesting area of study involves observing traits often associated with addiction, like high novelty seeking and impulsivity. Dagher and Robbins describe what happens to patients with Parkinson's disease when they abuse their medication (2009). The "Parkinsonian personality" has been characterized as rigid, introverted, and slow tempered well before the onset of motor symptoms. Often, a history of tobacco and alcohol abstinence is also noted, and generally there is a low incidence of drug addiction. Parkinson's disease is characterized by a deficiency in dopamine levels, with treatment including dopaminergic medications (drugs that increase dopamine). In some instances, these medicated patients suffer side effects of high dopamine, which have included compulsive behaviors like compulsive gambling, hyper sexuality, and even abuse and addiction to their Parkinson's medications.

From a psychological perspective, Khantzian and Mack have described "the heavy reliance on chemical substances to relieve pain, provide pleasure, regulate emotions and create personality cohesion" (1994). They have described this process as "self-governance"; and while no specific "addictive personality" may be identifiable, the maladaptive personality functioning in addiction creates a need for a cohesive sense of self and strategies to enhance self-governance capabilities that rely on substances for that purpose.

It would be unrealistic to think that deficits in the neurochemistry and reward circuitry in addiction, such as dopamine synthesis, would not influence personality functions in addicted patients. It has been speculated that these same circuits evolved in the brain for purposes of social attachment and are activated in addiction (Insel 2003). It seems logical that the strong connection that can occur between sober addicts plays such a pivotal role in addiction recovery. Conversely, those disorders that disrupt these attachment and affiliative systems, such as borderline personality disorder (Stanley and Siever 2010), can pose significant challenges in the treatment of those who have addiction complicated by these disorders. In all probability, there are adaptive styles that occur at different times in the addictive process. Prior to the addiction, a deficit in reward capacity could create a feeling of deprivation, leading to craving states and mood instability. This would certainly be the case, in an exaggerated way, during active addiction and withdrawal or craving states. During active substance use, exaggeration of previous temperament styles will certainly be present, and as a result of the ongoing addiction, character development would be arrested.

**Narcissism and Addiction**

Narcissism includes the exaggeration of one's self-importance and lack of empathy with others. This self-centered and typically defensive posture is inherent in the progressive nature of addiction. If the addict has preexisting narcissistic deficits, these deficits will be exaggerated in the addiction. If there is no history of them, the active addiction will create them since addiction turns the self against itself. The narcissism that accompanies addiction in any case has a narrative associated with it. The way we talk to ourselves is critical in determining our moods and behaviors. As previously discussed in this book, being on automatic pilot only perpetuates the habitual nature of the damaging choices chronically made in active addiction. In recovery there are opportunities to examine the way we talk to ourselves and get some distance from and restructure this inner dialogue.

The more unhealthy the personality, the more "fixed" is this sense of self, and consequently the more identified (or fused) this self is with feelings and thoughts. In the book *Healing the Healer* (1998), the authors address the issue of "the addictive personality." Much has been made of this addictive personality being suffused with narcissistic deficits, particularly those deficits that target problems with self-regulation. In his *Analysis of Self* (1971), Heinz Kohut identified a bipolar self (that is, two often opposing aspects of self) comprised of a self with grandiose ambitions and a self with idealized goals. These two poles are separated by a tension arc that is greatly amplified with disruption in either of these poles. If someone did not have proper mirroring in childhood because of abuse or neglect, the grandiose self would be diminished. Similarly, if there are continued difficulties in having role models, disruption occurs with idealized goals. The end result is disturbances in self-regulation, which of course is inherent in addiction. The difficulty in determining whether these narcissistic deficits helped cause the addiction or were caused by them demands a careful history and diagnostic interview. I do not believe there is a single "addictive personality" that is premorbid (prior) to addiction. As we describe later in this chapter, there are multiple configurations of temperament and character that contribute to active addiction and functioning in recovery. In any case, problems with self-regulation, self-awareness, and self-monitoring will invariably be problematic in addiction and potentially in addiction recovery (Kohut 1971).

Narcissism blocks the ability to successfully tolerate discomfort: moving away from preoccupation with self, enhances resilience that leads to more mature and reflective choices and decisions about how the fluid self will evolve. Frankl states "being human is being responsible—existentially responsible, responsible for our existence." Frankl discusses the interface between the existential vacuum of human existence and the resulting search for meaning and states that "what man actually needs is not a tensionless state but rather the striving and struggling for a worthwhile goal, a freely chosen task" (Frankl 1959).

## A Quantum View of Personality

On the tiniest, or "quantum," level of reality, things get very interesting. Minute particles get tangled and distances can disappear. What happens to one thing can affect another at a great distance, like a butterfly flapping its wings in Indonesia may result in a tornado in Kansas. As the great physicist Heisenberg proposed in his uncertainty principle, at this tiny level of reality, we change things by simply observing them (Heisenberg 1930). In fact, subatomic particles on this level of observation exist as waves or particles, actual clouds of uncertainties, depending on how they are observed.

Can this play out in the mind, in our very consciousness? Many think so. Much of the electrical activity of the brain that generates thoughts, feelings, and behaviors seems to be largely unconscious, beneath the level of our conscious mind. Often referred to as the "dark matter" of the mind, this is called the "default mode network," and it comprises 80 percent of the energy used in the mind (Boly et al. 2008). This network seems to have tremendous influence on our conscious thoughts and actions (Van den Heuvel et al. 2009). No wonder we typically return to a set of thoughts, feelings, behaviors, and personality adaptations. The set points may well be embedded in this murky dark matter of our minds. The electrical activities of the brain, as measured by EEG, seem to behave like weather patterns; that is, they are subject to clusters (called "strange attractors") that cause self-organization. These patterns, as described in chaos theory, are not completely predetermined. Chaos and quantum theory as applied to the mind create great possibilities for change—even in thought patterns that determine the often habitual ways of our personality (Zohar 1991).

> **Default Mode Network**
>
> This persistent level of background activity, below the level of awareness, represents the brain's "dark energy"
>
> Orchestrates systems (e.g., memory) for future conscious acts

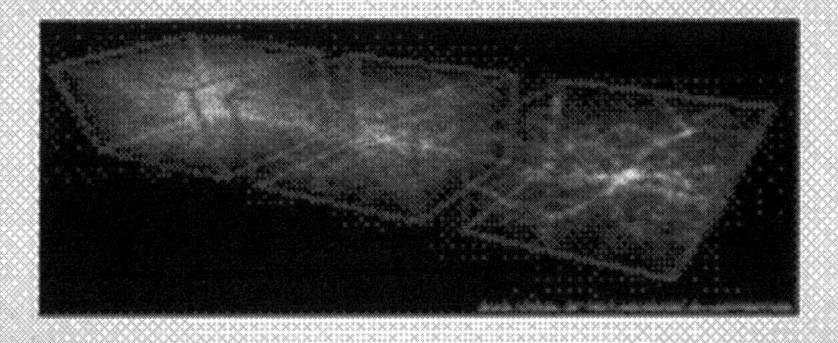

This would come as no surprise to Freud, who saw the profound role of the unconscious on our lives. Now experiments are showing that we can predict behavior by tracking this dark energy of the mind. Can we influence this hidden energy? If we apply the ideas of quantum entanglement, uncertainty, and chaos theory, perhaps we can even influence something as complex as personality and some of its hardened patterns more than we think. Today, pioneers (e.g., UCLA's Dr. Jeffrey Schwartz) are applying these principles in certain conditions like severe obsessive compulsive disorder patients with great success. By using the power of mindfulness to quietly observe their own behaviors, these often terribly disabled patients are getting better and neuroimaging of their brains show the changes they've made (Schwartz and Begley 2002).

## Positive Sobriety

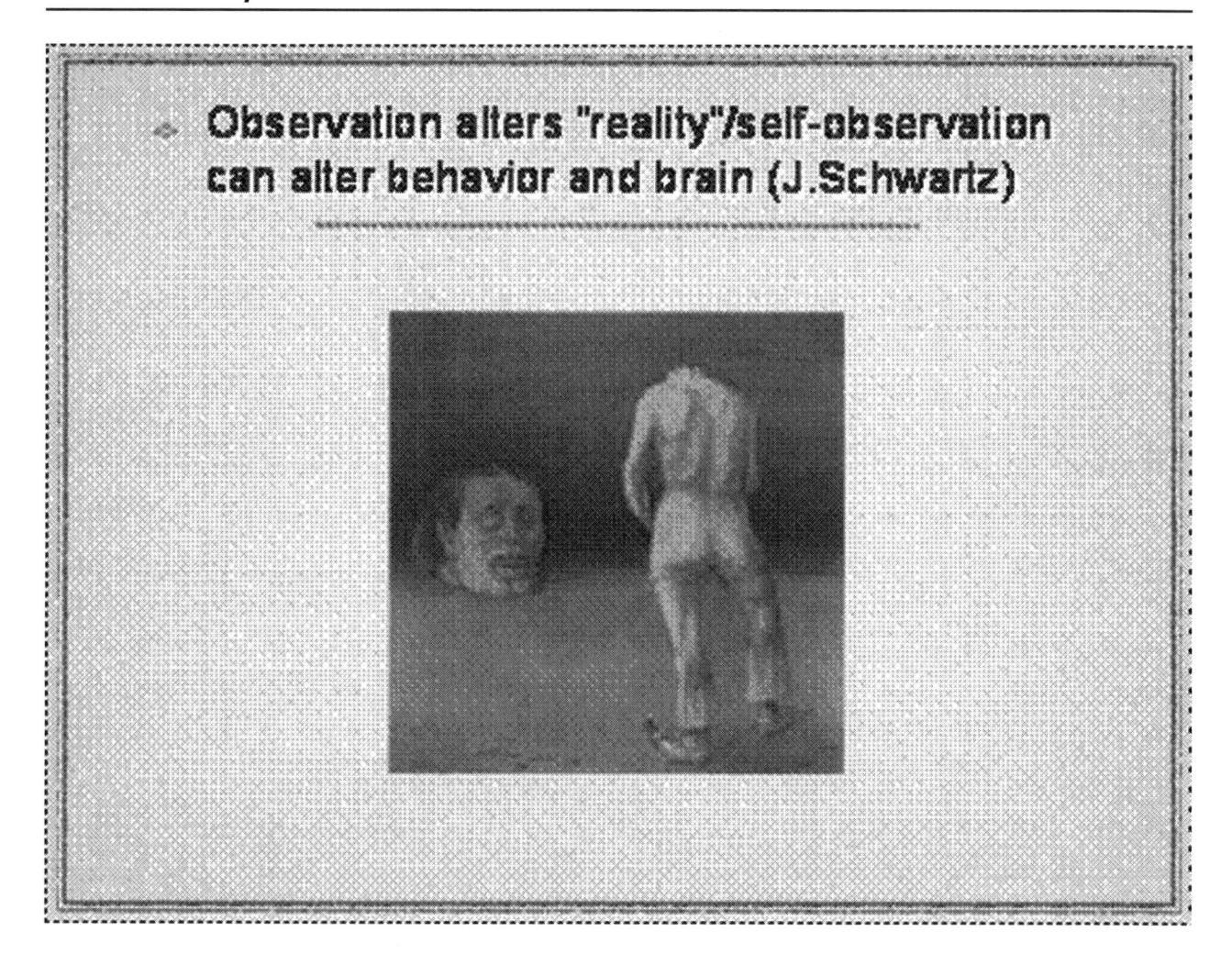

> **Observation alters "reality"/self-observation can alter behavior and brain (J. Schwartz)**

So we do not have to be slaves to this dark matter, not automatons blindly returning to a set point of self-defeating behaviors. If we can learn to quiet the mind and observe, we can change even something as fundamental yet ephemeral as personality. No easy task, but we have some tools to do this now that our active addiction is not calling the shots. Sometimes this can occur quickly, like with a spiritual insight. But even if this does occur, consistent change comes from deliberate effort over time. Understanding our history and feedback from small group sessions, individual therapy, and AA are essential. Self-reports like the BFI (see below) and the Millon can help provide a deeper level of insight into our personality styles, and of course, so can working the steps of AA. With the right kind of effort and help, we can observe those often elusive defects, and small changes of even one or two of the right ones can cascade and change the whole of who (we think) we are.

**Working to Understand Our Unique Personalities**

Despite how illusory our sense of self may be, our personalities have a tremendous influence in our lives. We become who we think we are. In some ways, our personality is of our own making. This gives us the freedom to change. Personality was defined by Allport in 1937 as "the dynamic organization within the individual of those psychophysical systems that determine his unique adjustments to his environment." In other words, "personality" refers to relatively stable patterns of thinking, feeling, and behaving, which can and do change over time. In fact, whereas it was once widely believed that personality traits never changed after a certain age, researchers are beginning to find that personality traits actually change across the lifespan and into old age. How do we know the structure of personality? More than 15,000 words in the English language have been identified that describe personality. A large amount of research that has asked people to sort personality words into different categories has consistently yielded five broad personality dimensions, typically referred to as the "Big Five" (more on this below). This finding has been replicated in many different countries and using many different languages. So, while there is a good chance that other personality traits outside of the "Big Five" exist, this widely adopted model of personality is a good place to start.

Personality greatly influences how we adapt to any given situation in an ever changing internal and external environment. Although our personalities change in response to so many factors in our lives, especially during active addiction, there are certain aspects of our unique personalities that are part of who we are. We can think of this as a personality "set point." This set point is where we return after any disruption in our lives. Some aspects of personality are in our DNA and other aspects are shaped as a result of our early life experiences and circumstance. Some of our personality adaptations are quite positive, but others are destructive. Within a positive sobriety mind-set, understanding our personalities in depth, our positive and negative dimensions, allows us to optimize our lives and chances for a continued recovery from addiction. As we will see, much of our work in treatment and twelve-step recovery is about uncovering these strengths and weaknesses and learning ways to change our personalities for the better.

Certain problems with impulsivity or overall poor coping skills within a personality structure can occur as a result of problems in early development. However, determining the relationship between personality and addiction can also be somewhat confusing since addiction can create deficits in personality; that is, addiction can interfere with the way people see themselves, cope with stress, and interact with other human beings. The relationship between personality and addiction becomes a chicken-and-egg problem that sometimes cannot be completely solved until someone is sober for an extended period of time. Learning about one's personality structure, especially as one moves away from the gravitational pull of the addiction, is essential.

The problem with personality is our tendency to be blind to certain aspects of it. Our sense of self is so variable and enigmatic that this should come as no surprise. It is these blind spots, or fatal flaws, as the ancient Greeks called them, that keep us stuck—that keep us repeating destructive behaviors and that keep us from being the best we can be. But if we can do the work on this path of self-awareness, we can identify and often change these stubborn self-defeating parts of us. In fact, by observing these defects, we have already opened the door to change. This is critical work we must continually do if we are ever to live happy, sober lives.

## The Big Five Personality Inventory (BFI)

There are a number of questionnaires that measure the "Big Five" personality trait domains (Goldberg, 1993). Most of these questionnaires are well-validated and are highly correlated with one another and they may also give us information as to our vulnerabilities to addiction (Belcher, Volkow 2014). When we talk about personality, it is common to ask if, for example, someone is an "extravert" or an "introvert." While this is a common way of thinking about personality, researchers now think of personality traits along a continuum. What this means is that while *all* people share the same personality traits, what makes us unique is *how much* of each trait we have. Think of it as a personal mix or configuration. For example, rather than ask if someone is an "extravert" or an "introvert", we may instead ask them "how extraverted (or introverted) are you?"

The Big Five model of personality consists of the following domains. Words in parentheses are those that are commonly used in association with each personality trait:

**Neuroticism** (negative emotion, anxiety, vulnerability, irritability)
**Agreeableness** (altruism, empathy, cooperation, politeness)
**Conscientiousness** (organization, industriousness, diligence, constraint)
**Extraversion** (positive emotion, enthusiasm, sociability, assertiveness)
**Openness/Intellect** (imagination, intelligence, curiosity, creativity)

**Hint: one easy way to remember the Big Five personality trait domains is by remembering the acronym "OCEAN."**

Openness- Refers to how creative, intellectual, and open a person is to new ideas. Individuals high in openness seem to be flexible in thought and are open to learning new ways of doing things.

Conscientiousness- Refers to how organized, self-disciplined, and persistent a person is. Individuals high in conscientiousness tend to be hard-working, punctual, and detail-oriented.

Extraversion- Refers to how talkative and outgoing a person is. The opposite of extraversion is introversion. Individuals high in extraversion tend to be more talkative and thrive in social large gatherings. More recent research is finding that higher levels of introversion has its own benefits, such as the tendency to be more introspective and perform well in academic settings.

Agreeableness- Refers to how warm, kind, and connected a person is to those around them. Individuals high in agreeableness tend to be well-liked by others and are likely to help others in need.

## 5. Who Are You? Personality and Addiction

Neuroticism- Refers to how anxious, temperamental, and moody a person is. Neuroticism is commonly referred to as the "maladaptive" personality trait, as individuals high in this trait tend to overreact emotionally, experience negative emotions frequently and intensely, have difficulty coping with stressful situations, and have a lot of emotional "ups" and "downs" throughout the day.

Psychometric research has demonstrated that five broad domains (the "Big Five") can be used to organize most aspects of personality. These traits tend to endure over time but can be modified with certain efforts.

Theoretically, most stable observable individual differences in cognition, emotion, motivation, and behavior fall into one of these five domains or can be described in terms of a combination of two or more of them. Personality research conducted on twin subjects suggest that both heritability and environmental factors contribute to the Big Five personality traits.

Twin studies suggest that heritability and environmental factors equally influence all five factors to the same degree (Bouchard 2003). Among four recent twin studies, the mean percentage for heritability was calculated for each personality and it was concluded that heritability influenced the five factors broadly. The self-report measures were as follows: openness to experience was estimated to have a 57% genetic influence, extraversion 54%, conscientiousness 49%, neuroticism 48%, and agreeableness 42%.

In the workbook section in Chapter 9, you will be given an opportunity to take a brief big five inventory to give you a sense of where you may fit in these categories. It is helpful to know this information so to be more aware of personality oriented triggers. For example, if you are high in negative emotions, it can create increased risk for relapse. By being aware of our individual traits or tendencies, we can change them over time, including being more positive. For those in the Positive Sobriety program, you also will have an opportunity to take a more extended personality inventory called the NEO.

### Plainly Stated

**Personalities are complex and unique. They are affected by our active addiction, during which our most dysfunctional personality styles are exaggerated or distorted. Although there is no addictive personality, the effects of the disease of addiction on our personalities influences our personalities even into our sobriety. Problems handling stress and rejection can be more present in addicts even in solid recovery. The good news is that in sobriety, we can be present enough to know what our unique vulnerabilities are and that even small changes can lead to bigger ones over time. In many ways we are who we think we are, and we behave accordingly. Thru personality inventories like the Big Five and the Millon we can better understand our personality styles and as we observe and understand our thinking and behavior, we can change.**

# The Millon

Originally developed by Theodore Millon, PhD, in 1977, the Millon Clinical Multiaxial Inventory (MCMI or "the Millon") is now on its third edition and has been translated into many languages (*MCMI-III*, Millon 1997). The MCMI-III is a validated and highly reliable personality assessment tool that has been utilized in a variety of settings with many specialized populations throughout the world. We use it in our treatment setting in conjunction with other clinical data such as interview material, patient history, behavioral observations, and other tests to inform clinicians of a patient's personality dynamics to help both the clinician and the patient better understand how those underlying dynamics impact substance use and vice versa. The MCMI started with a theoretical focus on behavioral principles of reinforcement and conditioning. Now, the instrument incorporates an evolutionary theory, meaning that personality is based on the tasks one confronts throughout life to exist, adapt, and reproduce. This describes a more dynamic approach to personality development while including interpersonal, cognitive, and biological influences and allows for a broader and more comprehensive understanding of the etiology of addiction. The goal of personality assessment is to determine which aspects of personality shape and constrain behaviors. As such, even individuals with the same diagnosis can exhibit different characteristics.

Millon and colleagues (2004) discussed personality disorders as resulting from a combination of predisposing and precipitating factors. Examples of predisposing factors are heredity, socioeconomic status, habits resultant of early trauma, and family atmosphere. Precipitating factors are clearly demarcated events, such as a severe accident or death of a loved one, that trigger the underlying pathology present because of the predisposing factors. Also of relevance are biological factors, including gender

Many factor models of personality have been developed over the years (e.g., Costa and McCrae 1989; Clark 1990; Harkness and McNulty 1994; Tellegen and Waller 1987). Some contemporary factor models adhere to the personality constructs described in the DSM in terms of disorder; some are loosely correlated to the DSM and more rooted in theory.

The Millon is a personality inventory that we have found very useful in our clinical practice. This test has some elements not readily found in the Big Five and works very well with it as a supplement and cross-reference tool. The Millon has validity scales that are woven into the report so that under- or over reporting is factored into the diagnosis. The Millon tends to "pathologize" when describing axis II (personality) syndromes; that is, it describes personality adaptations in their most maladaptive mode. It also categorizes these adaptations in DSM terminology. This is useful as it can illuminate specific vulnerabilities under duress and assist in diagnostic categorization. The dialogue in the Millon regarding axis II pathology is particularly insightful and helpful to get to the core of some of the patients' behaviors and thinking patterns. The Millon is designed to be interpreted by a doctorate-level clinician and is never given to the patient.

**Plainly Stated**

**The Millon is a very useful personality inventory. It is designed to show the most vulnerable personality adaptations and needs to be interpreted by a doctorate-level clinician. It is most useful in guiding clinicians in planning treatments.**

# 6. What Are You Looking For?

There are many reasons addicts engage in their addiction, even after a period of sustained abstinence. We previously discussed the disease aspect of addiction, emphasizing the power of reward, or "magical connection," as well as eventual deficits in memory, learning, and decision making. In addition, problems with mood, boredom, and painful feelings play a triggering role in addiction. Khantzian (1997) has written extensively on his self-medication hypothesis. He made a compelling argument that addicts often have difficulty with intense feelings and their regulation. He observes that addicts experience their affects in extreme: they feel too much, or they feel too little or not at all. Recognizing these addicts' inability to put feelings into words, Khantzian noted addicts often suffer with vague discomforts with relationships, self-esteem, and feelings of emptiness they are barely conscious of that can drive their addiction. This difficulty with feelings can combine with the disease of addiction to create the need to self-medicate these uncomfortable feelings. Khantzian described how the properties of certain substances can specifically interact with an addict's particular problems with certain feeling states. For example, opiates have been known to reduce feelings of anger and rage (often not consciously experienced) in some addicts. This is in part because of the pharmacologic properties of opiates. Therefore, addicts with difficulty in dealing with anger may gravitate to opiates as a drug of choice. Similarly, stimulants like cocaine can counter boredom or intensify pleasurable experiences in those addicts prone to those types of feelings. Alcohol and other sedatives can improve self-esteem and help overcome shyness because sedatives can reduce social anxieties and feelings of emptiness. Other drugs and addictive behaviors (e.g., sexual compulsivity, overeating, gambling) can "self-medicate" a number of feeling states, states of mind, and sensory experiences. It is critical that there be continued vigilance regarding these states. As recovery evolves, one can relax and trust intuition as a guide. However, a life of sobriety will always require a certain degree of vigilance and reflection, and as such, an addict needs different strategies in early and longer-term recovery.

There are a number of theories regarding craving states and why addicts return to use after a period of abstinence. Newton and colleagues (2009) review five such theories: negative reinforcement ("pain avoidance"), positive reinforcement ("pleasure seeking"), incentive salience ("craving"), stimulus-response learning ("habits"), and inhibitory control dysfunction ("impulsivity"). The Newton study, whose human subjects were methamphetamine addicts, found that the greatest number of respondents (56 percent) stated pleasure seeking as the reason for use, followed by 27 percent stating impulsivity as a primary motivator.

In the Dutch article "A Three-Pathway Psychobiological Model of Craving for Alcohol" (1999), Verheul and colleagues separate craving into "reward craving," "relief craving," and "obsessive craving" and pair each state with an underlying neurotransmitter system: reward involving dopamine and internal opioids, relief involving GABA, and obsessive craving involving serotonin. This study placed an emphasis on medication strategies targeting the underlying neurotransmitter process.

The following descriptions emphasize the return to use following some stable period in sobriety, hence the assumption that there is some distance from the "gravitational pull" of the disease. The longer one is in recovery, the more evident the motivation to use can become-if one carefully explores this motivation. It is also important to consider the reactive patterns that lead to craving often 'cue induced' (like seeing the bar you always drank in) as we discussed in the disease section.

# Early and Longer-Term Recovery

### Early Recovery

We define early recovery as the first year of abstinence and working a program of recovery. Remember, abstinence alone will not facilitate positive sobriety.

It is often said in twelve-step circles that participants should make no major decisions in the first year of recovery from addiction. As with so many observations made in the program, scientific inquiry substantiates this observation. The damage done by addiction can be observed in tests like the SPECT study illustrated below that shows the disruption of oxygen addiction can cause.

## 6. What Are You Looking For?

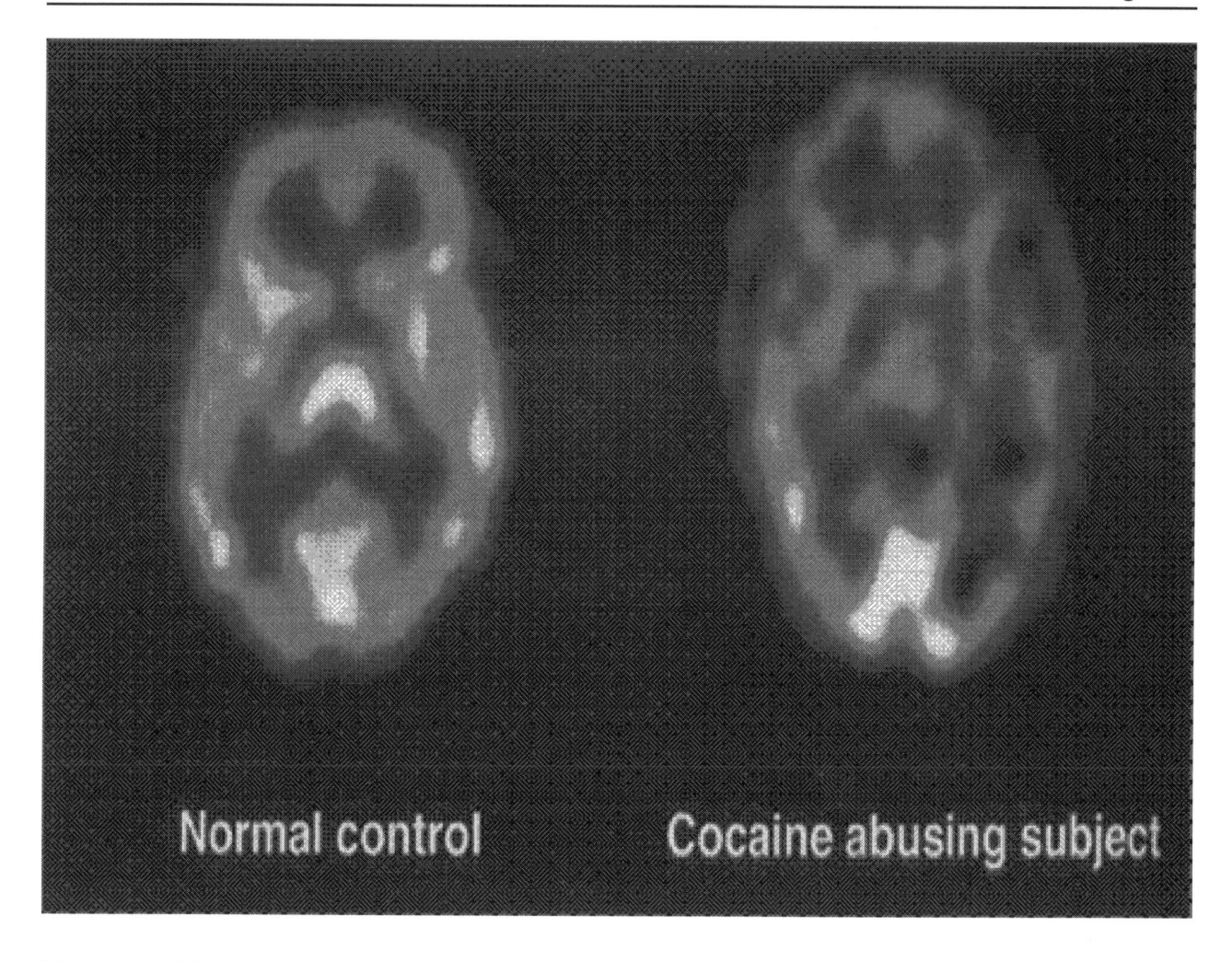

**Normal control**     **Cocaine abusing subject**

**This SPECT study shows a normal blood flow pattern on the left. The brain on cocaine shows multiple areas of black, representing compromised blood flow. (Kaufman 2001)**

The first few weeks of abstinence are particularly difficult even after the detoxification period (see "Post-acute Withdrawal Syndrome (PAWS)" in chapter 4 for further information).

Addiction can cause permanent brain damage, but this damage is the exception. In chapter 1, we discussed the three stages of addiction and said the third stage is a potentially permanent change in how the brain processes reward (specifically, how it synthesizes proteins). The brain has enormous regenerative properties. This includes "plasticity," or the ability to create new pathways and heal damaged ones. But the brain needs time to heal from the assault of addiction. Over time this occurs in most abstinent people. Working a program, like going to twelve-step meetings, meditating, and exercising, will facilitate and accelerate this brain-healing process.

**Positive Sobriety**

The healing addicted brain can then accommodate a central element of positive sobriety: improved decision making. The ability to choose is what addiction compromises and recovery facilitates. This is not only about choosing to use or not. It is also about the ability to choose how we live our lives, how we think, act, and feel. Recent research has suggested that there may be a predisposition in decision-making capability along with an inherited "reward sensitivity" in the addict. In their research, these authors suggest that addicts also inherit some of their reactive tendencies to cues (that substances make worse), a state often referred to as "cue reactivity".

The importance of moving away from reactive patterns, or "automatic pilot," cannot be overemphasized. We know through studying posttraumatic stress disorder that traumatic memories get stored in the limbic (deep emotional) areas of the brain. When these memories are triggered, they are processed much faster than our reflective ability to process what is really happening. This is similar to the reactive, automatic responses involved in addiction. So, we need to buy time for the brain to heal and provide greater capacity for reflection. The strategies used in treatment and provided in this book will help with that.

## Longer-Term Recovery

After approximately a year of abstinence and recovery, the strategies to enhance reflectivity can become more natural to us. This allows for refinement of these efforts with often greater benefit. Here, the question, "What am I looking for?" may be more subtle. With greater reflective capacity, there is increased ability to move beyond a predominately biologically driven process to a deeper psychological and spiritual one. One needs to ask, "What am I looking for?" in greater depth. This involves some discernment between states of mind, body, emotion, and spirit.

## States of Mind

Later in this book, there is an expanded discussion of the challenges of certain thought patterns and the importance of mindfulness and being present. Negative self-talk is a frequent trigger for use.

## States of Body

Acute or chronic physical pain is a complex problem when it is present in addicted individuals and requires a separate discussion. However, typical somatic (bodily) discomforts can be a trigger for use. Careful reflection on what we are physically experiencing can create the space for healthy and effective responses. Somatosensory treatments are particularly useful for somatic expressions of psychic pain that are seen with a number of disorders like depression and especially trauma.

## States of Emotion

Being in touch with feelings is arguably one of the most important efforts in addiction recovery. Reflection can identify often poorly identified or even unconscious feelings.

### States of Spirit

The need to transcend our states of mind, body, and emotion is universal. We have observed that addiction can sometimes be a misguided attempt at transcendence. It is no coincidence that alcohol is referred to as spirits!

### Plainly Stated

**The disease of addiction explains a lot of about why we use the way we do. But there is much more complexity in this than meets the eye. Our unique personality styles and responses to stress of all kinds are critical to understand if we are to engage in a positive sobriety. As time in recovery increases, so can our awareness of our unique triggers and responses.**

### 1) Rush

Looking for the intensity of the Rush is common with use of many substances and many addictive behaviors. Freebasing cocaine is a classic Rush experience. It is typically brief, intense, and highly rewarding, leading to a strong need to repeat the experience. If the addict pairs the cocaine use with reinforcing behaviors like sex or gambling, this will intensify the Rush experience. Other stimulants like methamphetamines or inhalants provide the same intensity. Other substances can be used in a way that creates Rush-type experiences. For example, consuming large amounts of alcohol in a short time and injecting drugs like heroin provide the Rush experience. Many addicts get addicted to the Rush of the needle alone as much as the drug being injected.

### 2) Buzz

This is a more subtle experience that is less intense and longer in duration then the Rush experience. Alcohol, more slowly consumed, creates the typical Buzz experience. Marijuana and some designer drugs like ecstasy also fit into this category. Many substances used together can prolong the experience, like combining stimulants with alcohol. Common reasons someone seeks the Buzz are to facilitate connection with others or to deal with social isolation.

### 3) Comfort

Using the addiction to seek out Comfort is universal in addictive disease states. It may be a primary trigger or accompany other motivations, but it is typically present in some form. The addiction itself creates the need for Comfort when the addict attempts to self-medicate the negative side effects of the addiction such as withdrawal. Most substances and rewarding behaviors have a potential to relieve or Comfort us. Sedatives like Xanax are specifically designed for this purpose and are commonly abused. Virtually all substances, including alcohol, pain killers, and even stimulants (in paradoxical responses), can have this comforting effect. Rewarding and comforting behaviors like compulsive sex and compulsive overeating can have the same effects as addicting substances. Chronic pain conditions are often a primary motivation for seeking Comfort and relief in addiction. Difficulty sleeping is a frequent trigger for comfort oriented substances.

## 4) Energize

The need to find a source of stimulation is ubiquitous in our culture. Coffee and tea are universally used for this purpose. Although in high amounts caffeine can be addicting, stimulants like Ritalin and Adderall are more typical agents used to enhance energy levels. And while these agents can help treat conditions like attention deficit disorder, they are highly abusable and typically contraindicated in addicts.

## 5) Making a Statement

There are times when the addict is not seeking a particular experience when they use. Engaging in the addiction can sometimes be a way to make a statement, like "I am tired of my life and give up" or "I need to get out of this marriage or job, but I don't know how." In using the addiction to make a statement, the effect is not what is primarily motivating the use. A desired effect is secondary to the conscious or unconscious goal of making a statement. Often, the lifestyle surrounding the addiction becomes comfortable and familiar to the extent that the addict does not want to give it up. This lifestyle can provide a sense of meaning and purpose for the addict that can overshadow the destructive course that may be obvious to even the addict. For example, the efforts made to obtain the drug (or object of an addictive behavior) can become ritualized and reinforcing in themselves. Additionally, at the end of these efforts, a predictable reward is always at hand. Despite the pain and suffering of this lifestyle, the addict can lack the motivation to change, since change requires work and the rewards of a sober lifestyle are not as immediate or predictable. At times the addict will identify with a hedonistic lifestyle like "sex, drugs and rock and roll" as a way to attempt to elevate their self-esteem and excuse their excesses.

The statement an addict in this scenario makes is, "Recovery is hard; I'd rather wallow in my addiction."

# Other Ways to Find What You Are Looking For

If one is aware of what they are looking for they can create options and alternatives to engaging in their disease. However it is critical that there be a concerted effort to avoid triggers. It is very difficult to manage certain triggering situations, especially early in recovery. We know this from the studies on cue-induced craving (for example, seeing a picture of the drug) discussed in the disease section. So we start with *avoidance*.

## Avoidance

Avoidance of triggers is one of the most important strategies to prevent craving-induced discomfort and relapse. This can be as elaborate as changing the workplace setting; for example, a nurse who diverted opiates from the workplace would no longer dispense controlled substances. It may be more subtle, like avoiding going to a wedding early in recovery.

We once had a patient who, despite serious efforts in sobriety, kept relapsing on alcohol. After a careful analysis, it became evident that he had been driving by the bar he used to frequent on his way home from work. Although he did not enter the bar, it gave him an uncomfortable feeling as he passed by it. And the cumulative effect appeared to contribute to his relapses. After changing his route, he is now many years sober.

Another patient realized that visiting his grandmother, who had several narcotic painkillers in her medicine cabinet, was a potential trigger. By having a plan, including bringing someone in recovery with him when he visited her, he was able to avoid a potentially dangerous situation. We must remember that reactive patterns stem from deep emotional memory and can trump our best efforts at making good decisions.

Sometimes we cannot avoid triggers; they are plentiful in the world we live in. They can occur in dreams in which we use, be present despite our best avoidance strategies, or simply spontaneously arise. This is why having these next three strategies are essential for a positive sobriety.

## Substitute

If you can identify what you need, you may be able to find a way to reproduce what you are looking for through nonaddictive means. For example, if the goal is to feel connected with others, one can call a sponsor or go to a meeting. If one is looking to free oneself from negative self-talk, a mindfulness meditation can help. Substituting for the Rush experience is most challenging. Sometimes recovering Rush addicts find healthy ways to generate this experience, such as engaging in competitive sports or high-risk activities like sky diving or rock climbing. The Buzz is easier to substitute. Many nonchemical coping skills like meditation, exercise, and connecting with others can produce a sustained experience. The same is true for those seeking the Comfort effect from substances.

## Tolerate

There are many times when alternatives or substitutions are simply not possible. Learning tolerate discomfort is a critical part of recovery. In her book *When Things Fall Apart*, Pema Chodron emphasized that the very times we are distressed are often the times we can grow in awareness (1997). One needs to learn to *be* with discomfort and allow that experience to guide one more fully into being OK with what is. The compulsive need to continuously change what one is experiencing often underlies craving states. Cultivating the capacity to *be* with discomforts can be transformative.

## Transcend

Mindfulness, meditation, and prayer are effective ways to fulfill the very human hunger for transcendence. In this case, the intent is not to substitute or tolerate but to observe what is motivating them in a nonjudgmental meditative state. This is perhaps the most evolved way to deal with addictive drives.

## Plainly Stated

**We must always be diligent in avoiding triggering situations, but there is no way to completely avoid them. There are several ways we connect with our drugs of choice to satisfy a certain need, especially early in the addiction when we perceive a benefit. What we are looking for may be a rush, buzz, to energize, to receive comfort, or to make a statement. It can have one particular effect or a combination of a few or all of these experiences. These needs may stem from genetics, personality, or coexisting processes like an anxiety disorder, but they constitute real needs that we need to openly identify and acknowledge. Answering some simple questions in the worksheets in chapter 9 can help illuminate how this works for us and allow us to find healthy alternatives in our recovery. This allows us to get these needs met in healthy ways, including substituting, transcending, or sometimes learning how to just tolerate a temporary drive.**

## *PERSONAL PERSPECTIVE*

*I once had a sponsor who had spent time studying homeless people, some of whom were addicts and alcoholics. A popular saying among them was "getting off the natural." It meant that anything that would change their current state of being was to be aggressively pursued, even if they were in a relatively good place. Because of their limited resources, they sometimes drank rubbing alcohol or ingested similar toxins that would invariably produce sickness or worse. Anything was better than reality. One could argue that these people had little to live for or to celebrate in their lives. However, this is a common occurrence in this disease. I could relate to the need to feel anything other than what I was experiencing at the depth of my disease, even if it meant feeling worse. How curious it is to me now that going more deeply into reality, into what* is, *through meditation and mindfulness produces such peace and at times even bliss.*

## *DHA*

# 7. What Makes You Happy?

Ultimately, if people could learn to be helpless, could they also unlearn it? Could they learn to be happier? These questions led to the field of positive psychology: a discipline that influenced the idea of moving beyond simple symptom reduction to strategies of well-being and happiness, a way someone can learn from their painful experiences to grow in well-being and happiness. The concept of learning here is essential; we have the ability to learn certain things about ourselves and to put some things in place that can lead to greater well-being and happiness. This is how our path of recovery can be a clear path to well-being.

The elements described in this text focus on a sense of well-being and happiness in recovery. As mentioned earlier, a great deal of research has been done over the last thirty years regarding happiness and well-being. In summary, what makes people happy has less to do with the idea that happiness can either be quickly achieved or bought and more to do with long-term satisfaction. This may require rethinking your beliefs about the nature of happiness.

Instead of equating happiness with pleasure or fun, it is more beneficial to think of happiness as a state of contentment, one that has less anxiety and regret, and certainly one that is absent of addiction and addictive behaviour. It is also important to recognize that brief periods of pleasure, although important, sometimes stick out as what really leads to happiness. However, remember that human beings habituate to both pleasure (the hedonic adaptation principle described earlier) and pain, and for that reason, intense pleasure can never last. This is true whether it comes from achievement, wealth, fame, beauty, possession, or from the addiction high. AA recognized the false promise of alcohol as it is related in the twelve and twelve, where we were "lost in the dust of what we thought was happiness." Ben-Shahar (2007) discussed the concept of happiness in terms of attitudes and behaviours that affect the present and the future in either a beneficial or detrimental way. He broke them down into the following four possible quadrants with four corresponding attitudes:

1) Present benefit/Future detriment = Hedonism

2) Future benefit/Present detriment = Rat Race

3) Future detriment/Present detriment = Nihilism

4) Present benefit/Future benefit = Happiness

Per these distinctions, one who falls into the hedonism category exhibits behaviors that bring instant benefit or gratification without extending into the future and that may even defy future benefit. The rat racer is constantly looking and planning for future benefit to the exclusion of the present. The nihilist is entrenched in the belief that their present unhappiness is their destiny and so pursues neither present nor future benefit; a belief that "People are mean life is hard and then you die." Happiness is possible when one modifies behavior to both satisfy present needs as well as work toward future goals.

Martin Seligman, certainly one of the pioneers of the field of positive psychology, has reworked his concepts of happiness (*Flourish* 2011) by looking to the concept of well-being. Happiness has traditionally been determined by surveys that measure someone's current mood, and the gold standard for measuring happiness was life satisfaction. In his 2002 book *Authentic Happiness*, Seligman described three elements of happiness: positive emotion, engagement ("flow," as described later in this chapter), and meaning. In his more recent analysis, Seligman adds two other elements: positive relationships and accomplishment. Together, the five elements constitute **PERMA: P**ositive **E**motions, **R**elationships, **M**eaning and **A**ccomplishment. He further emphasizes: the importance of freely choosing any given path and having the choice of this path one follows come from within. As was previously mentioned earlier in this book, Lyubomirsky (2008) described that 50 percent of our ability to be happy appears to be hardwired genetically, 10 percent is a matter of circumstance, and 40 percent depends on one's efforts in cultivating happiness. Ultimately, letting go, connecting with others, and doing the next right thing will move you toward a positive sobriety. The efforts you make in the following areas of character development (relating with self, others, and the transcendent) will facilitate this process. Having character development will allow the path of well-being to come from within.

The following ten elements reflect what create well-being in most people:

1) Self-acceptance, Taking responsibility

2) Optimism and gratitude

3) Goals that support a sense of Meaning and Purpose

4) Forgiveness

5) Kindness

6) Increased connection with family and friends

7) Mindfulness

8) Doing the next right thing

9) Flow

10) Spirituality

## 1) Self-Acceptance, Taking Responsibility

*Do not fight and reject or judge. Accept who you are and let go of all your struggles. It is less tiring and less of a strain, but it is not at all indifference.*

—C. R. Cloninger

The concept of letting go is critical to being on the path of well-being and sobriety. The word *surrender* is used frequently in recovery circles. Letting go includes the concept of surrender, which in turn requires a degree of humility and an understanding of the consequences of one's disease. However, letting go cannot really occur until one knows in some depth what they are letting go of. Letting go can be detrimental and escapist, a form of giving up, if one is not increasingly self-aware.

Self-awareness in addiction starts with taking responsibility and not blaming the addiction on others or circumstances. This self-examination and acceptance of the addiction is the first step of AA.

Much of recovering from substance abuse involves learning about yourself in your addiction and beyond it. Cloninger (1994) described the importance of listening to the psyche. He stated that this is a means by which we understand insight and can work with informed intuition: "The process of growth and self-awareness requires the purification of rational intuition by the mind becoming aware of itself."

Taking responsibility and not blaming others is the essence of the first step of AA: "We admitted we were powerless over alcohol and our lives had become unmanageable." According to Cloninger, self-acceptance and taking responsibility reflect hope. Hope, essential for positive change and well-being, also includes a sense of optimism and having a sense of meaning and purpose and setting goals.

## 2) Cultivating Optimism and Gratitude

*Our ancestors experienced their adaptive successes by engaging in a lot of the negative that we see in our lives today: the tendency to compare ourselves to others, striving for perfection, and the difficulty in forgiving and only having brief periods of happiness.*

—Baker et al., What Happy Women Know, pg. 14

Baker, Greenberg, and Yalof noted that evolution seems to favor negative rather than positive thinking. As a matter of survival, our ancestors were on high alert with anticipatory worry. They developed "mind machines" that were like Velcro for negative thoughts and Teflon for positive ones. Since our minds still operate with much of the same hardware as our ancestors, we all have to work at cultivating positive thinking and an attitude of optimism (2008).

Optimism can allow one to see problems as opportunities for growth. In addiction recovery, it is important to constantly learn how to grow as a consequence of the disease. For example, even craving can be instructive by allowing one to go more deeply into oneself to promote awareness of where the craving is coming from, to reach out to others to avoid the feelings of isolation that contribute to and exacerbate addictive behaviors, and to connect with a higher power to help one through the process.

Included in cultivating optimism is the concept of gratitude. Having gratitude shifts our focus to the positives in our lives and is associated with well-being (Emmons 2007).

The second step of AA states, "We came to believe a higher power could restore us to sanity." The insanity referred to in this step includes a clinging to negativity and cynicism. Insanity in other arenas has been described as repeating the same behavior and expecting different results. Incredibly, addicts often seek out addiction to create a positive experience or to become comfortably numb. While this may be happen, it does not come without consequences. The insanity is thinking the addiction exists without these consequences, or thinking that the addiction is the solution—that there are no other options to living. Choosing recovery begins the process of confronting that insanity and learning other tools to manage your life. In our sobriety we can learn to choose more positive thinking and associate with other people in recovery who support a sense of optimism.

## 3) Goals that support a sense of Meaning and Purpose

*I imagine that intention is not something you do but rather a force that exists in the universe as an invisible field of energy.*

—Wayne Dyer

Critical to the idea of goal setting is the concept of intention. The difference between intention and setting goals is simply that intention includes having goals but letting go of the outcomes. This is consistent with the third step of Alcoholics Anonymous, which is about "turning it over." For one individual, it may be turning it over to God, and to another, it may be simply turning it over to how things play out in the constantly evolving universe. Either way, there is openness to recognizing that the path one is on toward certain goals is more important than the outcome itself.

In the article "Ignite the Flame of Intention" (*Science of Spirituality* 2009), Largman described the power of intention: "As I distinguish it, the key difference between a goal and an intention is attachment. With goals, there is a fundamental belief that there is a logical path to follow, perhaps even a path that must be followed if you are to get from Point A to B." According to Largman, following a path works in the attainment of goals to a point, but intention is the mysterious energy that seems to oil all of our efforts with the sense of ease. With goals, people can be obsessed with following the steps necessary to attain them and being in control to make things happen, while intention allows for a more natural flow.

Intention in goal setting is absolutely vital to a deepened sense of meaning and purpose. It is equally critical, however, to recognize that the achievement of a goal or a series of goals will not in and of itself bring sustained happiness. It is particularly common for professionals to think that the next achievement, be it academic or economic, will bring them sustained happiness. However, if in the process of achieving goals one does not find pleasure, then the goals are invariably fantasies of future happiness. Once one has attained a goal and received gratification for reaching it, one quickly adapts to that fleeting gratification and begins to look for the next achievement to bring happiness.

Wiederman (2007) described that some people may be more prone to linking happiness to the achievement of goals than others. He described a continuum of nonlinkers to strong linkers. The nonlinker, on one extreme, does not think of any achievement bringing happiness, on the other extreme, the strong linker always connects some future achievement with happiness. The problem with strong linkers, Wiederman proposed, is that they tend to be obsessively focused on meeting a particular goal. Until they meet these goals, they are in a state of some degree of worry or anxiety and pressure rather than enjoying the pursuit of the goal. Research suggests that strong linkers are relatively less happy than other people during the process of pursuing goals because they feel that their happiness will be reached only after the goals are achieved. Again, the idea of habituation or adaptation plays a major role, so strong linkers will go from one achievement to another, hoping that the next achievement is what brings them sustained happiness and well-being. Have goals but with a sense of intention that provides meaning and purpose to our lives and that is not only dependent on a specific outcome.

## 4) Forgiveness

*Few people have been victimized by resentments than we alcoholics.*

—*Twelve Steps and Twelve Traditions,* p. 90

Everyone has at some point been involved in an incident with another person whom they felt hurt or wronged them either emotionally or physically. A range of emotions have the potential to arise from those experiences, but often these feelings reflect the victim's desire for retaliation or revenge or to avoid the transgressor altogether. The transgressor could be a stranger or someone with whom you are intimately connected. It is when these situations occur in intimate relationships that the work of forgiveness is often the most difficult. However, holding grudges and exhibiting behaviors to seek revenge upon or to avoid the person do not bring feelings of satisfaction and happiness; in fact, the opposite tends to occur. Resentment has often been described as someone swallowing poison and anticipating the pain in another individual, which refers to the truth that holding on to those kinds of negative feelings hurts you more than it does the object of your resentment.

Forgiveness does not necessarily mean forgetting, and there are times in which the transgression is beyond forgetting In many situations, however, the purpose of forgiveness is to let go of resentment and, if possible, recognize your role in any challenging or destructive relationship.

As true as it is that you have been the victim of a transgression, it is also true that you have transgressed another. Forgiveness does not necessarily mean not acknowledging the pain you've caused others or the pain that others have caused. It's not about becoming a doormat in the process. Rather, it's about examining the situation closely and making a conscious decision to move on. People often find that as they become better at forgiving others, others also find it easier to forgive them. In this way, relationships can be repaired and strengthened.

## 5) Kindness

*Positive affect promotes not selfishness or compliance-but a tendency to be kind and fair to both self and others...*

-- *Handbook of Emotions*

Practicing acts of kindness has been correlated with an increase in well-being. Researchers Williamson and Clark (1989) noted how helping others, through volunteer work, for example, improved mood and self-esteem. The twelfth step in AA involves helping other addicts and alcoholics. This is often referred to as a selfish step since the helper benefits as much as, and sometimes more than, the recipient, and many AA members will endorse the statement that no satisfaction has been deeper and no joy greater than from a twelfth step well done. Participating in a treatment program that emphasizes a therapeutic community framework provides a multitude of opportunities to practice kindness with peers.

## 6) Increased Connection with Family and Friends

*What I and others mean by the Great Story is humanity's common creation story. It is the 14 billion year science-based tale of cosmic genesis—from the formation of galaxies and the origin of life, to the development of consciousness and culture, and onward to the emergence of ever widening circles of care and concern.*

—*Michael Dowd*

Dowd (2008) described the limbic brain as what that represents "the inherited proclivities of our paleomammalian brain that include our deep drive to be in bonded nurturing relationships, and to acquire and retain high status in our social groups." This concept of brain development as represented in evolutionary psychology helps us understand why it is that accountability or the lack of it is the single best predictor of long-term integrity in individuals and groups. Mirror neurons are scattered throughout the brain and appear to have developed for the purpose of providing the hardware for empathy, the ability to grasp another's inner world. Dan Siegel describes how this neural capacity provides for endless implicit (rapid, often unconscious) messages to pass between people; language is only one way for communication to occur. We are wired to connect with others. Even slight variations in one's tone can trigger a fear response in the amygdala or a warm release of oxytocin (the connection neurohormone).

Improving relationships with others is a primary focus of positive sobriety and recovery. Within these relationships with others typically lies our greatest joy as well as our greatest pain. The majority of the steps of Alcoholic Anonymous and other twelve-step programs relate to relationships with others. Having greater intimacy with friends and family is a positive outcome in recovery. To sustain recovery, you need a community that values and elevates sobriety. Within that community, friendships will naturally flourish. These are friends you make in the program and at meetings. You may not necessarily always socialize with them, but a strong connection binds you. As is often said at AA meetings, "You may not like everyone here, but you will love them in a special way." There is a unique bond that occurs among those pursuing sobriety. In the program and at twelve-step meetings, there is an honesty and humility that binds members. The benefits of friendship and social supports are woven into the positive psychology literature. In more than one hundred empirical investigations, social support has been tied to reduced risks of all kinds, affecting both the likelihood of the initial onset of illness and the course of recovery among people who are already ill (Seeman 1996). Translating these connections to our most intimate relationships like those with our spouse and children can be the most satisfying of all our relationships.

## 7) Mindfulness

*When you are present, when your intention is fully intensely on the Now, Being can be felt, but it can never be understood mentally.*

—Ekhart Tolle

Mindfulness does not only include a meditative state, but also involves the idea of not "overthinking." Our normal waking consciousness is often in a mode of judgment. We may be judging our present experience, others, or ourselves. We are often lost in the past or projecting into the future. Most potentially damaging is the habit of judging oneself in comparison to someone or something else. Some believe that this process of overthinking and comparing ourselves to others is a major factor inhibiting our ability to achieve well-being. A counterattack for overthinking is being present, and it is also the antidote to hedonic adaptation. In other words, if you are present, you do not judge your experience or compare it with something past or anticipate something different in the future; you can be with whatever you are experiencing right now.

The ability to enjoy the journey, as when attempting to pursue certain meaningful goals involves learning how to cultivate the simple pleasures that occur in the moment. This can be done in a number of different ways and is an aspect of mindfulness, meditation, and the ability to be truly present, especially with one's senses. You can even convert a simple meal into a highly pleasurable experience if you take the time to savor it. Meditation is something that can always be further developed. You can work on cultivating this meditative capacity by practicing the techniques in chapter 8 of this manual. The eleventh step in AA, "We sought through prayer and meditation to improve our conscious contact" supports meditation.

## 8) Doing the Next Right Thing

*These [standards] are rules of conduct that we believe we ought to live up to regardless of the approval or disapproval of parents or any authority, and even when we do not feel empathy for those with whom we interact. Our moral standards are sustained by our imagination—because we can foresee that living up to them will bring about a more ideal world.*

—Schulman, 2005

Why does anyone stay sober? To avoid more pain and consequences? Or because they feel better sober? Certainly both of these motivations are factors for ongoing sobriety. Ultimately, though, ongoing sobriety requires an altruistic mind-set. That is, working a program and staying sober coincides with how one wants to live as a moral being. Addiction is harmful to oneself and invariably to others. Beyond pleasure and pain lie one's core values and principles driven by conscience and higher consciousness. Doing the next right thing from a deeper spiritual source within us is the foundation for ongoing abstinence and a happier life; in other words, a positive sobriety. Step 6 in Alcoholic Anonymous states, "We were entirely ready to have God remove all these defects of character." Willingness to change is at the very root of leading a life of meaning and purpose. Consider this and the implications of your role as co-creator in the evolutionary process and in the very evolution of consciousness. Michael Schulman, in his chapter "How We Become Moral" in the *Handbook of Positive Psychology* (2002), describes three moral systems: empathy, moral affiliations, and principles. He described empathy as being able to put oneself in another's psychological place. He believes empathy is a natural inclination that one feels particularly toward those who most approximate oneself. The moral affiliations system describes the process of identifying with those whom one feels are "good." Children internalize these models that then serve as guides for their behavior. Principles are basically rules of conduct instigated by imagination for the goal of bringing about a more ideal world rather than gaining praise or disapproval. One's self-esteem becomes tied into how congruent their behavior is with their principles. These three systems support each other.

Dacher Keltner from University of California, Berkeley, in his book, *Born to Be Good: The Science of a Meaningful Life*, describes how we are wired not only to connect with people but to promote the good in others. We evolved not only to survive by being self-serving but also to be altruistic—to benefit others, sometimes without personal benefit (Keltner 2011). Keltner refers to the concept of "jen," which Confucius developed centuries ago. It is the ability to acknowledge the good and bad in life and in this balance lean toward the good; he refers to this as "the jen ratio." This goes back to the dangers of nihilism and the importance of balancing present and future benefit previously discussed.

When certain brain structures, like the orbitofrontal cortex (critical for a sense of empathy) and its connections to the emotional brain and mirror neuron–filled parietal lobes, have not evolved (or are impaired, for example, due to early life trauma), this can lead to lack of empathy and even psychopathic behavior in some people.

In positive sobriety, the recovering addict can easily empathize with the addict who is still suffering, identify with others in sobriety and see sobriety as maintaining a personal standard of right and wrong. This personal standard of right and wrong can transcend both empathy and affiliations. So even if at times we may resent other addicts or our sponsor in AA relapses or for a period of time we just don't feel good, we maintain our sobriety simply because it is the right thing to do. We just do the next right thing. All of us have various strengths and weakness that are also in a state of flux as we respond to internal and external influences.

Step 10 in AA says, "We continued to take a personal inventory and when we were wrong, promptly admitted it," which reflects an ongoing effort to do the next right thing.

# 9) Flow

*A good life is one that is characterized by complete absorption in what one does.*

—*J. Nakamura, M. Csikszentmihalyi, Handbook of Positive Psychology, 2005*

The flow state combines mindfulness with creative pursuit. In the 1960s Csikszentmilhalyi and other University of Chicago researchers interviewed thousands of individuals to better understand the "flow state." They and others determined several factors that characterized this state, including intense and focused concentration on an activity that merges action and awareness; losing oneself in the process but maintaining a sense of control and mastery and finding the experience intensely rewarding, even independent of intended outcome; and often a loss of time. The flow state stretches and challenges one's capacities but does not overmatch existing skills and has proximal goals with consistent feedback. Flow can be experienced in work (for example, a surgeon immersed in a procedure) or play (like a runner being "in the zone"). It is the essence of enjoying the journey. And it utilizes and combines a number of the previous nine elements—mindfulness, letting go, goal setting, and even kindness and doing the next right thing when a flow activity has an altruistic component or end point.

The idea of being fully absorbed in a process that one finds interesting is defined as flow. A flow state would include something like being involved in a creative pursuit such as art or music. It can also mean being fully absorbed in something that one is doing that is meaningful. This can be as simple as gardening or as complex as doing surgery and includes all points in between. This underscores the importance of the balance between pleasure and meaning. Full involvement in the process is in itself a transcendent state where time seems to fly by (Csikszentmihalyi 1990, 1995, and 1997). Csikszentmihalyi and Seligman (especially in his most recent book *Flourish*) both seem to agree that the word "happiness" is overused and doesn't tell the whole story of optimal well-being. In a flow state, we don't notice happiness or pleasure because of our full absorption in the creative process.

There are no shortcuts to flow; one needs to work hard using the talents they have to be in flow. And happiness, or better stated, "satisfaction," can occur with the reflection on what was accomplished during the flow state. This satisfaction is greatly enhanced when the product of flow represents our values and can even contribute to the well-being of others.

# 10) Spirituality

*By Spirituality we mean here those issues of personal identity and transcendence that motivate people beyond the practicalities of daily living; these may be based on their religious commitment, but may also be defined more broadly, in terms of altruism, naturalism, or aesthetic ideals.*

— *Koenig*

The previous nine elements discussed are spiritual in that they transcend the practicalities of daily living as well as emphasize that critical balance between pleasure and meaning. Having spirituality has been noted by the vast majority of studies on positive psychology to be correlated with happiness and well-being (Lyubormirsky 2008). NYU's Mark Galanter and colleagues have shown the importance of having spirituality in recovery from psychiatric conditions as well as addiction (Galanter 2011). Having the ability to experience spirituality through transcendent practices like meditation is critical. Berkeley researcher LeeAnne Kaskutis studied spirituality in AA attendees and found that an experience of spirituality, not religious beliefs coming into the program, correlated with better outcomes. Putting spiritual beliefs like compassion and helpfulness into action is also invaluable for well-being. But also having a belief system of some kind, whether religious or secular, seems to complete the spiritual dimension necessary for well-being.

Beyond what one can do to influence positive outcomes, faith allows one to let go and accept that all is as it should be. Although twelve-step recovery involves relationships with self and others, spirituality is AA's primary emphasis. Along with meditation and, for some, religious involvement, AA provides a spiritual connection that is nondogmatic. One of the great contributors to the field of addiction, Jelinek, is quoted as saying, "Drunkenness can be a kind of shortcut to the higher life, the attempt to achieve a higher state without an emotional and intellectual effort" (Kurtz 1992). It is well-known by those in solid recovery that until the spiritual yearning within the alcoholic and addict is replaced with transcendent endeavors that lead to the discovery of a power greater than self and substances, replaced with other recovering people, and finally replaced with service for others also seeking sobriety, there can be no transformation. The Big Book tells its readers to "First of all quit playing God" (Alcoholics Anonymous, 4th edition, 2001, p.62). This act of surrendering involves a feeling of self-transcendence: the alcoholic is admitting they are no longer the center of the world and seeking a connection with a transcendent reality and with other people. The individual essentially stops playing God and starts seeking God (Cole and Pargament 1999).

## Plainly Stated

**In the positive psychology field, many studies have described what makes most people happy. These elements are common to working a program and mirror the twelve steps and promises of AA. Some of these elements may be easier to put into practice than others, but over time, we can get a sense of what we need to concentrate on as we progress in recovery. All ten elements described above are what the literature supports as necessary for well-being. As we progress in our recovery and identify our personality strengths and weaknesses and understand what we were looking for in the addiction (and healthy alternative ways to get there), we can define these elements for ourselves and pursue them in an organized and comprehensive way. This is true spirituality in action.**

# 8. Developing a Meditation Practice

## Meditation: The Antidote to Hedonic Adaptation

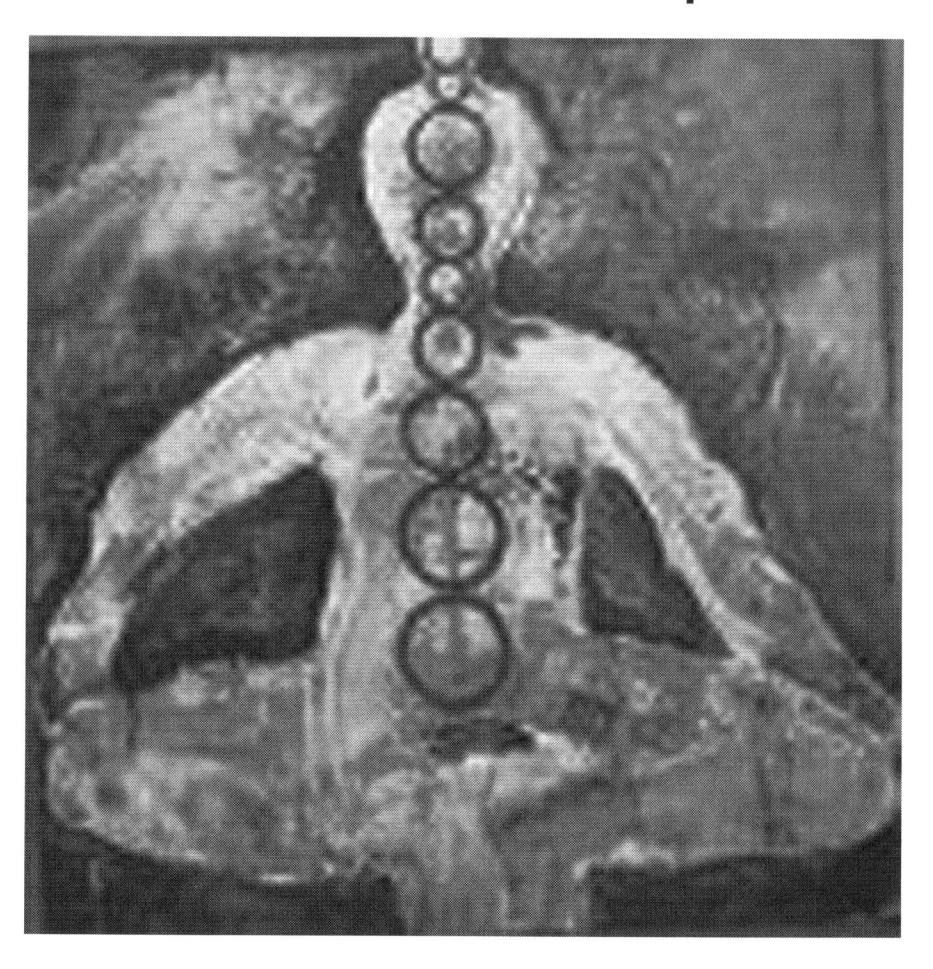

# Positive Sobriety

Positive sobriety includes abstinence from mood-altering addicting substances and addictive behaviors along with cultivation of the capacity for higher states of consciousness. This requires developing a routine of some kind of daily meditative practice that best suits your temperament and lifestyle and taking this higher consciousness from the practice space to the rest of your life. The challenge for any recovering addict is the ongoing potential for relapse into the addiction with all of its associated cravings and consequences. As discussed earlier, the disease of addiction has a neurobiological and psychological underpinning that can be called "the addictive drive" that can be quiescent in recovery but remains ubiquitous. That is why sober addicts are "in recovery" and never "recovered." This addictive drive, however, can represent a unique opportunity. When this drive presents itself in recovery in its various forms, such as craving or feelings of deprivation, these symptoms of the disease can remind us of the need to continue and even intensify our meditative practice along with our other recovery activities.

Through sublimation, the addictive drive can be fuel for transcendence. The sober addict can achieve and maintain these higher states of consciousness and the improved relationships with self, others, and a higher power that emanate from them. Your well-being and life can depend on it. This is a unique reinforcement and motivator with the ultimate gift of addiction recovery.

In his book *How God Changes Your Brain*, Dr. Andrew Newberg determined that just twelve minutes of a focused meditation demonstrated positive changes in key areas of the brain, including the prefrontal cortex and anterior cingulate. These changes suggested improvements in memory, mood, and attention and reduction in anxiety. In fact, imaging showed these changes occurred over just an eight-week period (2010). It would seem that making a commitment to a twelve-minute or longer daily meditation is easily accomplished, especially if someone is convinced that it will be helpful. Dr. Sarah Bowen and her team at the University of Washington under the direction of Dr. Alan Marlatt demonstrated the benefits of mindfulness meditation in reducing relapse (Bowen et al. 2009).

This chapter outlines several ways this can be achieved, since research and clinical observation suggest that different meditative practices exist for differing aptitudes. These various efforts find their commonality in creating enhanced moment-to-moment awareness, a higher state of consciousness or "presence." This effort would seem very achievable; however, my personal and professional experience is that this is not an easy task. Our busy schedules and myriad other resistances (especially our endless barrage of thoughts) can make this a greater challenge than even committing to a regular exercise regime. Nonetheless, this is an effort worth making.

For the sober addict, this simple yet profound practice can reduce stress and craving, improve mood, and even create a capacity for experiencing higher and ultimately profoundly rewarding states of consciousness. For addiction clinicians, incorporating mindfulness in their practice can be highly beneficial for both therapist and patient. Meditation is a disciplined approach to be "fully present." Mindfulness is paying attention in a particular way in the present moment nonjudgmentally. A regular meditation practice enhances one's capacity to live mindfully, which is a state of being that is highly compatible with recovery from chemical dependency as well as mood disorders and other painful states of mind.

# 8. Developing a Meditation Practice

Thinking allows human beings to transcend a purely instinctual state of being. However, our thinking patterns can become excessive and even compulsive. The idea is not to stop thinking but, by cultivating mindfulness, to think and act effectively when one needs to while being present more often. And when painful thoughts or feelings arise, mindfulness allows you to step back from and be identify less with these thoughts or feelings. Sobriety is not just abstinence. It is also the ability to tap into an expansive frame of reference for your feelings and states of consciousness. This in turn allows for an experience of openness and expansiveness we can choose at any time. "Normal waking consciousness" can be described as a state of "sleepwalking." Many people live out their entire lives in this state. Addiction represents an exaggerated unconscious state of being on automatic pilot. Unless a disciplined effort is made to transcend this sleepwalking, this state will most likely never change. People may temporarily "wake up" at different times, for example, by noticing the beautiful changes in nature during a crisp fall day or the filtering of sunlight through the trees on a clear day. For a brief moment, one may gaze upon these beautiful visions and experience being fully present. Although this higher order of consciousness is always available, practicing certain techniques makes it more regularly available (Newberg and Waldman 2010).

The vast majority of addicts do not come to treatment with an established meditative practice. The challenge then becomes finding a way to motivate these individuals and to impart some simple but effective ways to meditate. Once they establish a foundation in a basic meditative practice, people can have numerous ways in which to deepen and expand their practice if they so choose. The first step in this process is dealing with resistances. In our experience, many individuals, whether they struggle with addiction or not, have certain degrees of resistance to meditation. The following have been areas of resistance that commonly have to be dealt with in order to motivate an individual to cultivate this practice.

## Finding the Time

The single greatest obstacle that we've observed to cultivating and maintaining a meditative practice is simply finding the time in someone's busy schedule to do this on a regular basis. The minimum or optimal amount of time to meditate can be variable with 12 minutes a day often cited but others suggest a longer period of time (Benson & Wallace 1972; Mahesh Yogi 1963). Transcendental Meditation (T.M.) has contributed a considerable amount to the existing literature on the benefits of meditation, especially as it relates to our busy Western culture. T.M. recommends twenty minutes of sitting meditation twice daily. In his book *The Attention Revolution* (2006), Allan Wallace suggests a minimum of twenty-four minutes a day based on the percentage of a twenty-four-hour day that would seem minimally optimal for meditation. Kabat-Zinn (1994) uses forty-five minute modules in his mindfulness-based stress reduction course. There have been excellent books that address the time considerations in meditation and have espoused effectiveness in even briefer meditative practices. Refer to the references for a number of excellent books for further reading. This treatment program recommends that one commits a minimum of twenty minutes of meditation most mornings of the week. If someone has time for only five or ten minutes, then that is better than no time at all. Many recovering people in twelve-step programs do a daily morning reading as part of their recovery routine. Here one can simply devote a period of time after that reading for a more focused meditation. Also included in this chapter is a "traveling meditation" that can be done on one's daily commute. If you effectively learn to meditate and begin to see the benefit, you will find the time to continue it.

## Suspicion of "New Age" Approaches

Although meditation itself has been utilized in both Eastern and Western contemplative practices (by St. Augustine and in the traditions of the Kaballah and the Sufi, for example), many are suspect of the implications of a meditative practice. This approach is practical and secular. As one begins to evolve in their meditation practice, they may apply this to their own belief system or be involved in a more traditional religious practice. Here meditation is emphasized as a practical approach to balancing the mind, which then opens up a greater capacity for self-exploration, improvement of relations with others, and engagement in transcendent or transpersonal relations. It is important for each individual to decide for themselves the nature of their conceptualization of a meditative practice.

## Mental Clutter (Hyperactivity)

Most beginners in meditative practice confront hyperactivity, in which one is bombarded with thoughts, feelings, or sensations during their meditative practice. In regards to hyperactivity of thought, intrusions of physical sensations, and so on, it is recommended that without judgment, you simply observe what's going on and go back to the task at hand, be it observing the breath or focusing on a particular part of the body (as in the body scan). The idea is to have a back and forth between distraction and focused meditation.

## Fatigue (Laxity)

Becoming sleepy or spacing out during meditation is common at different times for anyone who meditates. Meditating in the morning can reduce the likelihood of this occurring. Sitting in an erect posture and avoiding meditating while lying down can also help. Some may need to keep their eyes open while meditating. The longer you meditate, the more alert and focused you will become.

## "Nothing Seems to Be Happening"

For many in the early phases of learning to meditate, there is often a distinct frustration regarding a perceived lack of benefit. Sometimes there is even frustration and self-condemnation regarding this lack of benefit. Here a parallel can be made to developing an exercise routine. Very often, people who have never exercised describe feeling sore and uncomfortable even with short periods of exercise. However, as they become better at exercise and more effective in their exercise practice, they can exercise for longer periods of time and realize greater benefit. This is true for meditation as well. Research has

## 8. Developing a Meditation Practice

demonstrated there are actually measurable changes in the brain that occur during meditation (Davidson et al. 2003). These changes appear to deepen as the meditator does it more and becomes better at it over time. In other words, stay with it.

**Meditation Can Be Isolative**

One of the single most dangerous conditions for someone with an addiction is isolation. One needs to be aware that anything can be abused. In fact, the addict's motto can be "anything really worth doing is worth abusing." There is a definite risk as someone cultivates a meditative practice to attempt to seek a "high" as the ultimate purpose of the meditation. This can lead to a self-centered and isolative practice. Although a sense of well-being and even euphoria can occur during an even limited meditative practice, this should not be the goal but only an appreciated side benefit. The ultimate goal in meditation is to provide greater balance in your relationships with self and others in a transcendent realm.

Regularly practicing an extended meditation such as a twenty-five- to forty-minute body scan or breathing meditation is a critical way to experience a still, mindful state. Capturing this state throughout the course of the day is essential to learning mindfulness in action.

# Stop, Look, Listen and Breathe"

STOP → Catch yourself in any activity (driving, especially while stopped in heavy traffic; waiting in line; just hanging out; or even watching TV). Really notice being caught in whatever activity you are engaged in. Then step back and take a few deep breaths.

LOOK → Really observe. Focus on what you are seeing. Notice the shapes and colors without necessarily defining them as "objects." Take in all of what you see in a nonjudgmental way. If your eyes are closed, notice the patterns you see in the darkness.

LISTEN → Be fully with what you hear. Notice the texture of the sounds. When someone is talking, take in the full content of what is being said or expressed. Be present with everyday sounds or music.

BREATHE → Let the senses of seeing and hearing be a gateway into being fully present. Notice your breath as you intensify these two sensory inputs. As you breathe, feel yourself in your body; perhaps in your hands you will notice a pulse. You're there.

In anticipation of or response to stressful events, the STOP, LOOK, LISTEN, and BREATHE exercise may be used. Applying this exercise to painful events (and the thoughts and feelings associated with them) allows for the creation of the space in which you can observe thoughts as thoughts and feelings as feelings and not be over identified with them. Choosing to be present rather than reactive is a victory in recovery.

# Meditative Aids and Approaches

**Yoga**

Yoga is meditation in movement. This ancient practice has a universal appeal and is particularly helpful for people who have a hard time turning off their minds. Many have observed that yoga is particularly helpful for people whose addiction is complicated by anxiety disorders, particularly those caused by past traumas, as seen in posttraumatic stress disorder (PTSD). Because yoga integrates mind, body, and spirit, it is usually helpful for everyone as long as a skilled teacher recognizes the various physical limitations each participant has. Research has examined the effects of yoga and meditation on PTSD. Brown and Gerbang (2005) highlight the positive effects of both yoga and meditation in the treatment of trauma, PTSD, stress, depression, anxiety, and substance use disorders. Benefits have been shown to be maximized both physically and physiologically through training with a skilled instructor and daily practice of thirty minutes in duration. Van Der Kolk (2006) found that exposure to extreme stress, such as that which may trigger PTSD, affects brain function. Since traumatized individuals are vulnerable in their reactions to sensory information, yoga and meditation may help attenuate the stress response and be beneficial to individuals suffering from PTSD.

**Biofeedback**

Biofeedback literally means using electronic equipment to feed back information reflecting the physiological effects resulting from changes in the mind. Many different techniques are used to find what is most effective for each individual, including breath training, visualization, autonomic techniques, EEG, word repetition, muscle relaxation, and body scans. Individual sessions are the best way for each person to learn and practice what works best for them. No two brains react in exactly the same way, so it is to one's advantage to try a variety of different techniques.

Biofeedback has long been utilized in the medical profession to manage chronic pain conditions, hypertension, addiction treatment, and insomnia, among others. In the mental health field, biofeedback is used to reduce stress and therefore stress-induced illnesses, to manage symptoms of anxiety, and to enhance a calmer and more focused state of mind. Biofeedback essentially involves teaching an individual to tune in to their physical, emotional, and mental states with an emphasis on prioritizing those states of being that are more adaptive. It is an active process requiring full participation of the individual. With practice, the person learns the most effective way to control their autonomic nervous system, thus disturbed bodily symptoms are brought under control by attending to the mind-body connection.

**Neurofeedback**

Neurofeedback is a type of biofeedback that utilizes a computer program to help guide an individual into a desired mind state. There is increasing support for the effectiveness of neurofeedback, particularly in improving attention both in the general population and those with attention deficit disorders.

The neurofeedback mechanism involves placing electrodes on the scalp corresponding to the areas of the brain that one wishes to examine and modify. These electrodes are then attached to a particular computer program that measures the brain wave frequencies in those particular areas of the brain. With the assistance of a neurofeedback technician, the computer program can then modify these brain waves. For example, a sound associated with a computer image can be used for this purpose. The sound and image modification subconsciously reinforce certain brain wave states by helping the trainee to be more present when entering into the desired brain wave state. Over the course of several training sessions that last thirty to forty minutes on average, the trainee can experience the desired change in brain states as evidenced by brain wave modifications. This has been described as "the tail wagging the dog." That is, our brain produces brain waves based on specific brain states such as being calm or focused. The idea of neurofeedback is to alter the electrical activity of the brain to then change the underlying affective states.

For the purpose of meditation, neurofeedback often utilizes what is called alpha-theta training, which induces a state of calmness. However, depending on the individual, it may be necessary to also improve attention and focus as well as calmness. This means training different areas of the brain at higher frequencies. We have found that neurofeedback can be an effective adjunct to a meditative practice. A recent and very effective and easy to use portable neurofeedback device called the "Muse©" uses a slim headband that measures brain wave activity providing feedback thru an app attached to an iPhone or iPad.

## Cardiac Coherence

Cardiac coherence describes a practice that synchronizes the heart rate and breath. This practice creates a peaceful state that also facilitates potential improvements in cardiac function. There are several devices that assist in this process. The emWave PC Stress Relief System© is once such tool. It allows you to monitor your heart rate on a screen in response to emotional states. The emWave operates on the premise that intentionally altering one's emotional state through focusing on the heart will in turn affect the neurological input from the heart to the brain. This works because respiration becomes more rhythmic and deeper when people are in a more positive emotional state, making the heart beat more rhythmically, which helps the body work more in sync (in physiological coherence). The goal is to train people to self-generate positive emotions for their rhythmic effects that then extend physiological coherence. This makes it easier for the person to sustain the rhythm and coherence even in the face of challenging situations and makes the person less susceptible to old physiological symptomatic responses such as anxiety and depression.

## Imagery and Positive Affirmations

There are increasingly more commercially available guided meditations on the market. The basic premise behind the guided meditations is to create a meditative environment for users to utilized in the privacy of their homes. These are particularly useful for people who require some assistance reaching that desired meditative state. In some cases, having a provided image or another's voice giving direction allows the person to focus on the meditation when they might have difficulty keeping the mind from wandering if left to meditate in silence. Repeated exposure to a more positive mind-set and to more positive thoughts can influence both the conscious and subconscious mind toward more positive thoughts, feelings, and behaviors.

## Prayer

The act of prayer has been utilized by a great majority of people for a very long time. It is an outlet for people to connect to a higher power and enjoy the feeling of talking to a loving and omnipotent entity that will hear them, lift their burdens, enlighten them, and heal them and others. It is not necessary to have a defined belief system for one to pray, but it does make it easier. There have been numerous studies that verify that the results prayer and meditation have on the brain are similar (Newberg and Waldman 2010).

## Audiovisual Entrainment

Like neurofeedback, these devices work with brain wave frequencies. As opposed to teaching patients to actively alter their brain waves, audiovisual entrainment devices use light and sound to subtly guide overall brain wave frequency into the desired range. These devices, like the David (see appendix C), involve glasses and earphones. The glasses have programmed strobe light effects and mixtures of frequencies that are described in a booklet that accompanies the device. The frequencies are audible. There are also commercially available auditory entrainment devices such as the Thompson recordings that have a subtly disguised frequency underneath a particular musical track to help guide the user into the desired state.

## Audio Brain Wave Entrainment (BWE) with Binaural Beats

To date, audio brain wave entrainment (BWE) with binaural beats has been most useful and easiest technology to use for our patients. Typical BWE works because its rhythmic pulses are able, at least to some degree, to attract the brain's neural firing rhythms into its own rhythmic train of influence. With BWE using binaural beats, the effect is greatly enhanced. With binaural beats, the right and left olivary nuclei (the audio-processing centers in the two hemispheres of the brain) work together in order to detect the phase difference between the two audio inputs. The brain creates and perceives a third, or "phantom," tone (the wavering sound) referred to as a "binaural beat."

# 8. Developing a Meditation Practice

> ## Binaural Brain Entrainment
>
> - Right and left olivary nuclei (the audio-processing centers in the two hemispheres of the brain) work together in order to detect the phase difference between the two audio inputs.
>
> - The brain creates and perceives a third or "phantom" tone (the wavering sound) referred to as a "binaural beat."

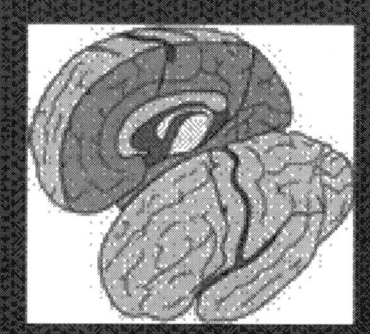

We have been using Hemi-Sync© technologies by the Monroe Institute, who have an array of commercially available CDs and training programs. We have an advanced Hemi-Sync trainer consulting with our program and have weekly binaural beat sessions. We are also using newer SAM© (spatial angle modulation) technology that allows for a Doppler effect and can be used with a speaker system as well as headphones.

There are different frequencies that are preset in the tapes we use that all have different effects. Here is a description of some of the frequencies used, typically mixed in with the guided meditations for maximum effect.

**Beta (13–39 Hz):**

- Sensorimotor awareness - Wide awake -

- Alert, focused. Analyze and assimilate new information rapidly.

- Complex mental processing. Peak physical and mental performance.

- Cannot be sustained indefinitely. Prolongation of beta can lead to exhaustion, anxiety, and tension. Short bursts of beta have been used for improving cognitive intelligence.

**Alpha (8–13 Hz):**

Accelerated learning. Beginning of drowsiness. Relaxed alertness. Zen meditation.

- "Open Focus" (term coined by Dr. Les Fehmi). Can stimulate the release of serotonin (vital in the regulation of mood and sleep).

**Theta (4–8 Hz):**

- Hypnogogic state. Dreaming sleep.

- Creativity, inspiration. Vivid imagery. Deep meditation. Out-of-Body experiences. Facilitating long-term memory. Spontaneous emotional release. Profound attitudinal and behavioral changes.

**Delta (0.5–4 Hz):**

- Deep, dreamless sleep. Formless/expansive experiences.

**Plainly Stated**

**Meditation is a powerful way to improve well-being. The many benefits include improved mood, more positive emotions, better decision making, and even better physical health. You only need to do twelve minutes a day to get these benefits, but for many people meditating is difficult, especially early in recovery. There are a number of resistances, but there are many ways to meditate and several aids to help us. It is well worth the effort to find what works best for you and to use it regularly.**

# Two Guided Meditations

*Both of these meditations (in conjunction with Bob Holbrook) have been carefully synchronized with binaural frequencies or SAM and are available at the Positive Sobriety website.*

## 1) Notice, Focus, and Feel

The following meditation involves three basic categories. It begins with noticing or mindfulness, then moves to focusing on guided imagery, and then goes to generating positive feelings (emotions). To notice, in a nonjudgmental way, is the hallmark of mindfulness meditation. Recent research suggests that mindfulness meditation involves specific parts of the central nervous system and specific neurotransmitters. Mindfulness appears to be mediated by the norepinephrine system and shifting the locus of neuronal activity from the right to the left prefrontal cortex that has been suggested to be correlated with positive emotions. Davidson and colleagues (2003) demonstrated that the left side of the prefrontal cortex is associated with awareness and positive feelings through their observations of brain activity in novice and experienced meditators. In coherence with attending to neuronal activity, the Notice, Focus, and Feel mediation first activates the left hemisphere during Notice, then activates the right hemisphere in Focus, finally integrating activity in both hemispheres during Feel. Purposeful activation of brain activity functions to reorganize and calm the brain through activation of neurotransmitters.

Focus meditations, such as those that involve guided imagery, seem to have an affinity for the dopamine system. You may recall that dopamine is responsible for facilitating reward (as in addiction) and is also active in the focusing of attention. If the focus then extends to surrounding areas, a feeling of being connected beyond the body can activate certain EEG patterns (specifically alpha-theta patterns). This is well formulated in the Open Focus mediations developed by Fehmi and Robbins (2007). In working with neurofeedback and monitoring EEG patterns, Fehmi and Robbins came across the powerful meditative states associated with including a sense of space in the use of guided imagery (2007). Additionally, imagery-induced loss of boundaries can create a right hemispheric dominance that can create a powerful transcendent experience. These observations were made by a neuroscientist who had a massive stroke in her left hemisphere (Bolte-Taylor 2008). This difficult situation created a right hemispheric dominance that was a path into these profound insights that continue to guide her spiritual life:

> My left hemisphere had been trained to perceive myself as a solid separate from others. Now released from that restrictive circuitry, my right hemisphere relished in its attachment to the eternal flow. I was no longer isolated and alone. My soul was as big as the universe and frolicked with glee in a boundless sea. For many of us, thinking about ourselves as fluid, or with souls as big as the universe, connected to the energy flow of all that is, slips us out beyond our comfort zone. But without the judgment of my left brain saying that I am a solid, my perception of myself returned to this natural state of fluidity. Clearly, we are each trillions upon trillions of particles and soft vibration. We exist as fluid filled sacks in a fluid world where everything exists in motion. Different entities are composed of different densities and molecules, but ultimately every pixel is made up of electrons, protons, and neutrons performing a delicate dance. (p. 69)

The feeling or emotion aspect of meditation has been well studied in regards to cardiac coherence. When feeling a positive emotion, particularly emanating from the heart, studies demonstrate that this improves cardiac coherence. Cardiac coherence is measured by the synchronicity between our breath and our heartbeat. As described in the cardiac coherence section, the more synchronized your heartbeat is with your breath, the greater the cardiac coherence.

## Notice, Focus and Feel Meditation:

- Notice

Spend five minutes simply noticing your breath. As you do so, breathe deeply as you inhale and exhale. You may notice your mind wandering. When you get caught in a thought or a sensation or a sound or any distraction, bring yourself back without judgment and simply notice the process as you go back and forth from your breath to whatever distraction grabs your attention.

- Focus

In this next five-minute period, focus your attention on your hands and fingers. As you relax during meditation, your blood vessels dilate and this actually creates an increase in your core temperature. Feel that warmth in your hands and fingers. As you exhale, concentrate not only on this warmth but on letting go.

- Feel

For this next five minutes, breathe into and out of your heart. Notice a sense of positivity emanating from your heart. As you exhale, send out positive feelings. These positive feelings can be to a specific person, a group of people, or even a higher power. You can also send those positive feelings back to yourself.

This meditation is set to binaural beats or SAM that go from alpha to theta (with a short period in delta) and is available on the Positive Sobriety website. This utilizes the research from Peniston and his group that showed good results in alcoholism using alpha-theta training. In addition to long-term (three-year year) abstinence rates of 80 percent, the Peniston Protocol has consistently produced the following very healthy personality changes (Penniston, 1993):

(1) Significant decreases in scales labeled schizoid, avoidant, passive-aggressive, schizotypal, borderline, paranoid, anxiety, somatoform, dysthymia, alcohol abuse, psychotic thinking, depression, psychotic depression, hypochondriasis, hysteria, schizophrenia, social introversion, and psychotic delusion.

(2) Significant increases in social warmth, abstract thinking, stability, conscientiousness, boldness, imaginativeness, and self-control.

Thus, the Peniston Protocol consistently produces positive changes in what many consider to be hard-wired aspects of personality. These dramatic personality changes enhance the patient's ability to cope without substance abuse, significantly reducing the likelihood of relapse.

The alpha component helps with focus and the slower theta and delta frequencies with letting go which may also mirror the "signature" that Dr. Andrew Newberg and his associates at the University of Pennsylvania obtained from looking at scans of practiced meditators (Newberg, 2010) . This signature showed heightened activity in the left frontal lobe (associated with attention and decision making) and lowered activity in the posterior parietal area (associated with letting go of physical boundaries). This is what I call a "focused letting go": a meditative state that is a combination of mindful awareness and attention that transcends our sense of self. This also is useful when we reflect on intention and goal setting in a way that has focus but a greater emphasis on journey than on destination.

**Body Scan**

Sit comfortably but with your back straight. If you are especially tired, lying down is fine.

1) Start with both feet. Notice the sensation in your toes, in the bottoms of your feet, and in the top of your feet. Stay with the sensation or even the lack of it for about a minute. Breathe into both feet, and then go on to ankles and calves.

2) Work upward in this manner, hesitating in breathing into each area: the upper legs (try to sense the femoral pulse), buttocks, pelvis, and hips.

3) Now move to the lower back and up to the middle and upper back. Then shift to the abdomen and then chest (feel the ribs, the expansion and contraction of the lungs, and the beat of the heart).

Now, starting at your fingertips, slowly work up the forearms, elbows and upper arms. Focus on the shoulders and neck (feel the carotid pulse).

4) Go to the face, jaw, lips, teeth, cheeks, eyes, and forehead. Then to the top of the head, the crown, and the back of the head.

5) Now imagine an opening about the size of a quarter on the very top of your head (like a whale's or a dolphin's blowhole). Breathe in through this opening to your hands and feet. Slowly push out the breath, letting go of any residual tension. Do this for about three breaths.

6) Try this body scan technique for about fifteen minutes, and then go directly to the breathing meditation described below.

**Positive Sobriety**

| | |
|---|---|
| Posture: | Sit with your back straight, chest out, and chin down. Imagine a string gently pulling up at the crown of your head. You can keep your eyes open, lids soft, and gently focus about three feet in front of you and about one foot down. Try to softly visualize as much of the room as possible. Let your eyes eventually defocus altogether. If it is more comfortable and fatigue is not an issue, keep your eyes closed. |
| Breathing: | Breathe through your nose. Let your inhalation fill your abdomen as well as your lungs. Breathe into your qi (that area about two inches below your navel). This is very centering. |
| Counting: | Silently say, "one" as you exhale. Let the number extend through the entire exhalation, and drop your head down to your chest, resting your arms and hands on your stomach. Hesitate at the end of the expiration and feel the energy of being still and present as you straighten up and inhale again. Go to "two" and continue through "ten." Then start again at "one." |
| Thoughts: | Thoughts will come up. Don't fight them. Label them like passing clouds and remind yourself to go back to the breathing and counting. |
| Sounds: | Listen to the sounds you hear. Pay attention to the texture of the sounds. Notice if the sounds you hear become distracting. |
| Body Sensations: | Pay attention to the sensations you experience in your body. What might these sensations be telling you? |
| Feelings: | Notice your emotions in response to meditation and being present in the moment. |
| Fatigue/Drowsiness: | Always go back to posture. Good posture keeps you focused. Remember, meditation is discipline. |
| Variation: | Go through all the above techniques but experiment with the following: When inhaling, imagine taking in your pain/discomfort and/or anyone else's and exhaling peace and serenity. This makes you a vehicle of healing and positive energy. |
| Routine: | We recommend a minimum of ten minutes of meditation each day followed by the body scan, preferably in the morning. |

# 9. Positive Sobriety Worksheets

The following explanations, questions, and answers in the following sections will assist you in learning about your unique personality strengths and weaknesses, what you were looking for in your addiction, and what brings you true satisfaction. These worksheets will help you through this journey of self-exploration.

## Who Are You? Personality and Addiction

The Mini IPIP (Donnellan et.al.) is a brief questionnaire that can give you some insight as to how you might score on longer versions of Big Five personality inventories. The following inventory is a modified version of the questionnaire.

Instructions: Below are phrases describing people's behaviors. Please use the rating scale below to describe how accurately each statement describes you. Describe yourself as you generally are, prior to your addiction. Describe yourself as you honestly see yourself, in relation to other people you know of the same sex, and roughly your same age. Please read each statement carefully, and then fill in the number (1-5) in the space next to each statement that most accurately describes you. Use the scale below to guide your responses.

**1=Very Inaccurate**

**2=Moderately Inaccurate**

**3=Neither Inaccurate nor Accurate**

**4=Moderately Accurate**

**5=Very Accurate**

**Positive Sobriety**

1. Am the life of the party (E)

2. Sympathize with others' feelings (A)

3. Get chores done right away (C)

4. Have frequent mood swings (N)

5. Have a vivid imagination (I)

6. Talk a lot (E)

7. Am interested in other people's problems (A)

8. Rarely forget to put things back in their proper place (C)

9. Am rarely relaxed most of the time (N)

10. Am not interested in abstract ideas (I)

11. Talk to a lot of different people at parties (E)

12. Feel others' emotions (A)

13. Like order (C)

14. Get upset easily (N)

15. Have no difficulty understanding abstract ideas (I)

16. Rarely keep in the background (E)

17. Am really interested in others (A)

18. Rarely make a mess of things (C)

19. Frequently feel blue (N)

20. Have a good imagination (I)

The letter in parenthesis after each question refers to one of the big five domains. For example, the question number 14 "I get upset easily" has (N) after it. This stands for Neuroticism. If you go back to chapter 5 and review the section on the "Big Five" you can get sense of your personality strengths and weaknesses. Neuroticism is the one score you want to be low in; the other 4 you want to be high in.

**Openness/Intellect**

1. Add up the scores for items 5, 10, 15, and 20 ____.

**Conscientiousness**

1. Add up the scores for items 3, 8, 13 and 18 ____.

**Extraversion**

1. Add up the scores for items 1, 6, 11, and 16 ____.

**Agreeableness**

1. Add up the scores for items 2, 7, 12 and 17 ____.

**Neuroticism**

1. Add up the scores for items 4, 9, 14 and 19 ____.

**Interpreting your scores**

For each personality trait domain, higher scores indicate higher levels of that particular personality trait. For example, a score of 20 on the neuroticism domain indicates a high level of neuroticism, whereas a score of 5 on the conscientiousness domain indicates a low level of conscientiousness. Scores for each personality domain ranges from 5 to 20.

Then answer the following questions:

1) What were your lowest and highest scores?

2) Can you describe how any of these traits may have triggered or protected you from addiction and relapse?

**Positive Sobriety**

3) What are some practical things you can do to better your scores? For example, learning to meditate to reduce your neuroticism score.

# What Are You Looking For?

As described in chapter 6, there are many reasons addicts engage in their addiction, even after a period of sustained abstinence. We previously discussed the disease aspect of addiction, emphasizing the power of reward, or "magical connection," as well as eventual deficits in memory, learning, and decision making. However, problems with mood, boredom, and painful feelings can play a triggering role in addiction. This worksheet can help you recognize your motivational pattern and assist in some practical strategies for ongoing recovery.

**Worksheet on the Five Specific Reasons to Use:**

The following questions can give you some insight into how your addiction appeared to assist you in certain areas of your life. Answer these in the context of when you felt your addiction worked for you. The following **five reasons to use** can be a guide to better understanding what you are looking for in your addiction. You may find that you relate to many or even all of these.

Answer the questions below using a scale of **1 through 5** to indicate which items are most or least applicable in your addiction.

Rate items below from **1** being **the least applicable** and **5** being **the most applicable** to you. You may need to do each section differently for different substances you have used. For example, cocaine may have provided a 5 in Rush and a 1 in comfort, and perhaps alcohol provided just the opposite.

1) **Rush**

   I often used substances (or addictive behaviors) to heighten my sensory experience of music, movies, food, sex, etc. . . . . . . . . . . . . . . . . . . . . . . . . . . . . . . . . . . . . . . . . . . . . . . . 1 2 3 4 5

   I often felt more intensely present in the moment when I was high. . . . . . . . . . . . 1 2 3 4 5

   I always go for the most intense experience any way I can get it . . . . . . . . . . . . . . 1 2 3 4 5

2) **Buzz**

    My addiction intensified or soothed my relationships . . . . . . . . . . . . . . . . . . . . . . . 1 2 3 4 5

    I seemed to get more work done and enjoyed work more when using . . . . . . . . . . 1 2 3 4 5

    I felt more confident when high . . . . . . . . . . . . . . . . . . . . . . . . . . . . . . . . . . . . . . . . 1 2 3 4 5

3) **Comfort**

    My addiction helped me cope with stress, anxiety, insomnia and/or physical pain . . . 1 2 3 4 5

    I hardly worried when I was under the influence . . . . . . . . . . . . . . . . . . . . . . . . . . 1 2 3 4 5

    My addiction made me less fearful . . . . . . . . . . . . . . . . . . . . . . . . . . . . . . . . . . . . . 1 2 3 4 5

4) **Energize**

    My addiction gave me the energy I needed to accomplish my goals. . . . . . . . . . . . . 1 2 3 4 5

    Getting motivated has always been a problem for me . . . . . . . . . . . . . . . . . . . . . . 1 2 3 4 5

    My addiction made my job/tasks much more interesting . . . . . . . . . . . . . . . . . . . . 1 2 3 4 5

5) **Making a Statement**

    My addiction made my life bearable. . . . . . . . . . . . . . . . . . . . . . . . . . . . . . . . . . . . 1 2 3 4 5

    My addiction provided a lifestyle that in some ways is hard to give up . . . . . . . . . 1 2 3 4 5

    My addiction seemed to give me a sense of purpose and meaning . . . . . . . . . . . . . 1 2 3 4 5

## Other Ways to Manage What You Are Looking For

Now that you are more aware of what you are looking for when you use from your answers above, you can create **new options** and **alternatives** to engaging in your disease. Often the same strategy may serve to substitute, tolerate, or transcend urges to use. A strategy like talking to someone, going to meeting, meditating, or exercising can provide different qualities of experience, all useful in

## Positive Sobriety

combating reactive responses and patterns. For example, talking to someone when seeking comfort may provide the same type of experience as a drug (substitute), may buy time until the stressor or craving passes (tolerate), or may allow you to rise above the situation (transcend). The last type of strategy can be very rewarding, as the stressful situation can be a vehicle to a deeper and more rewarding experience, like connecting with someone in a meaningful way. This is the essence of a positive sobriety when the gravitational pull of the disease creates an opportunity for a higher order experience. The best way to minimize reactive patterns, though, is reducing triggering situations by avoiding them.

### Avoidance

*Name some strategies that would minimize being triggered to use:*

### Substitute

*Name some ways you can substitute for the areas you scored the highest in:*

### Tolerate

*What can help you tolerate a craving or stressful situation?*

**Transcend**

*What kind of activities can you do to transcend a need for use?*

# What Makes You Happy?

These following ten elements were summarized in chapter 7:

1. Self-Acceptance, Taking Responsibility
2. Cultivating Optimism
3. Goals that support a sense of Meaning and Purpose
4. Forgiveness
5. Kindness
6. Increased Connection with Family and Friends
7. Mindfulness
8. Doing the Next Right Thing
9. Flow
10. Spirituality

Answer these questions to apply them to your present state of recovery:

1) Self-Acceptance, Taking Responsibility

*Describe one negative thing about yourself that you are currently accepting and taking responsibility for.*




2) Cultivating Optimism

*Can you describe something you are now optimistic about?*




3) Goal Setting/Meaning and Purpose

*Describe a recent goal in your recovery.*

## 9. Positive Sobriety Worksheets

4) Forgiveness

*Comment on someone you have recently forgiven.*

5) Kindness

*Describe a recent act of kindness.*

6) Increased Connection with Family and Friends

*Can you name and describe your connection to a recent friend in the program?*

7) Mindfulness

*How are you able to be more mindful today?*

8) Doing the Next Right Thing

*Give an example of when you last did "the next right thing."*

9) Flow

*Describe a recent event when you experienced flow.*

## 10) Spirituality

As stated in chapter seven, the nine elements above are spiritual elements. Ultimately recovery is a spiritual process and the following questionnaire is way to measure this. You can go back to these questions at different points in your recovery and see how your spirituality is changing over time.

The IPIP spirituality questionnaire (Goldberg et al., 2006), based on items from the Values in Action questionnaire (Peterson & Seligman, 2004), is a brief questionnaire that can provide some insight regarding your level of spirituality. This has been modified for our purposes.

Instructions: Below are phrases describing people's beliefs and behaviors. Please use the rating scale below to describe how accurately each statement describes you. Describe yourself as you generally are, prior to your addiction. Describe yourself as you honestly see yourself, in relation to other people you know of the same sex, and roughly your same age. Please read each statement carefully, and then fill in the number (1-5) in the space next to each statement that most accurately describes you. Use the scale below to guide your responses.

# 9. Positive Sobriety Worksheets

**1=Very Inaccurate**

**2=Moderately Inaccurate**

**3=Neither Inaccurate nor Accurate**

**4=Moderately Accurate**

**5=Very Accurate**

1. \_\_\_\_\_ Believe in a universal power or God.

2. \_\_\_\_\_ Am a spiritual person.

3. \_\_\_\_\_ Keep my faith even during hard times.

4. \_\_\_\_\_ Have spent at least 30 minutes in the last 24 hours in prayer or meditation.

5. \_\_\_\_\_ Am who I am because of my faith.

6. \_\_\_\_\_ Believe that each person has a purpose in life.

7. \_\_\_\_\_ Know that my beliefs make my life important.

**Scoring:**

1. Add the scores for items 1, 2, 3, 4, 5, 6, 7= \_\_\_\_.

Scores for this scale range from 7 to 35, with a score of 35 indicating a very high level of spirituality and a score of 7 indicating a very low level of spirituality.

**Key Websites:**

**Positive Sobriety**
The website companion to this manual
www.positivesobriety.com

**Online Information and Support Resources for Addictions**
National Addiction Hotline
1-800-993-3869
National Institute on Alcohol Abuse and Alcoholism (NIAAA)
www.niaaa.nih.gov

National Institute on Drug Abuse
www.nida.nih.gov/nidahome.html

Substance Abuse and Mental Health Services Administration
www.samhsa.gov

Addiction Treatment Forum
Reports on substance abuse news of interest to opioid treatment programs and patients in methadone maintenance treatment
www.atforum.com

Dual Diagnosis Website
Provides information and support for dually diagnosed patients
http://users.eros.com/ksciacca

**Positive Sobriety**

Focus Adolescent Services
Comprehensive source of information, resources, and support for teens and families online
www.focusas.com

Institute of Alcohol Studies
Information on alcohol and the social and health consequences of misuse and abuse
www.ias.org.uk

Learn-About-Alcoholism
Educational resources on multiple aspects of alcoholism
www.learn-about-alcoholism.com

Mental Health Matters
A directory of mental health resources, treatment options, and support services
www.mental-health-matters.com

National Council on Alcoholism and Drug Dependence
Local resources, family education, intervention, mutual aid and support, medication, and recovery stories
www.ncadd.org

Recovery Connection
Helps locate addiction treatment centers and drug rehabilitation programs
www.recoveryconnection.org

Web of Addictions
Facts about abused drugs
www.well.com/user/woa/

Eating Disorder Referral and Information Center
Provides information and help in locating treatment centers
www.edreferral.com

National Association of Anorexia Nervosa and Associated Disorders
Promotes healthy lifestyles and the alleviation of eating disorders
www.anad.org

National Eating Disorder Association
www.nationaleatingdisorders.org
Helpline: 1-800-931-2237

National Council on Problem Gambling
Information on gambling addiction and resources for help
www.ncpgambling.org

National Center for Responsible Gambling
Research, education, and awareness
www.ncrg.org

## *12-Step and Self-Help Resources Online*

Alcoholics Anonymous
The official AA website: includes meeting directories, information, and communication forums
www.aa.org

**International Doctors of Alcoholics Anonymous**
Link to meetings, information, and membership
www.idaa.org

Alcoholics Anonymous Meetings Online
Online twelve-step meetings
www.stayingcyber.org

Narcotics Anonymous
Information and meeting finder
www.na.org

Essence of Recovery
Twelve-step recovery support
www.essence-of-recovery.com

Nicotine Anonymous
Smoking cessation support
www.nicotine-anonymous.org

Al-Anon and Alateen
Information and meeting directories
www.al-anon.alateen.org

Adult Children of Alcoholics
www.adultchildren.org

**Positive Sobriety**

Methadone Anonymous
Support website
www.methadonesupport.org

Codependents Anonymous
www.codependents.org
www.coda.org

Food Addicts Anonymous
www.foodaddictsanonymous.org

Gamblers Anonymous
www.gamblersanonymous.org

Marijuana Anonymous
www.marijuana-anonymous.org

Overeaters Anonymous
www.oa.org

Sex Addicts Anonymous
www.sexaa.org

Sexual Compulsives Anonymous
www.sca-recovery.org

SMART Recovery
A non-twelve-step recovery program
www.smartrecovery.org

Sober Sources Network
www.sobersources.com

The Sober Village
www.thesobervillage.com

Anxiety Self Help
www.anxietyselfhelp.com

Center for Online Addiction
www.netaddiction.com

Recovery Life
Spreads messages of hope and strength for daily affirmation
www.recoverylife.com

Recovery Zone
Twelve-step resource guide
www.recoveryzone.org

Onsite Workshops
www.onsiteworkshops.com

## Meditation Resources and Suggested Readings

The Monroe Institute/Hemi-Sync
Website to access Hemi-Sync meditations and learn about binaural beats technology and meditation
www.monroeinstitute.org/hemi-sync/

*Just for Today: Daily Meditations for Recovering Addicts*
By Narcotics Anonymous (1992)

*Keepers of the Wisdom Daily Meditations: Reflections from Lives Well-Lived*
By Karen Casey (1996)

*Meal by Meal: 365 Daily Meditations for Finding Balance through Mindful Eating*
By Donald Altman (2004)

*8 Minute Meditation: Quiet Your Mind. Change Your Life*
By Victor N. Davich (2004)

*Deep Meditation: Pathway to Personal Freedom*
By Yogani (2005)

*Opening to Meditation: A Gentle, Guided Approach* (book and CD)
By Diana Lang (2004)

*Meditation: How to Reduce Stress, Get Healthy, and Find Your Happiness in just 15 Minutes a Day*
By Rachel J. Rofe (2010)

*Meditation for Beginners*
By Jack Kornfield (2008)

**Positive Sobriety**

*Quiet Mind: A Beginner's Guide to Meditation*
By Sharon Salzberg, Sakyong Mipham, Tulku Thondup, and Larry Rosenberg (2008)

*Your Present: A Half-Hour of Peace: A Guided Imagery Meditation for Physical & Spiritual Wellness* (CD)
By Susie Mantell (2000)

*Stages of Meditation*
By The Dalai Lama (2003)

*Insight Meditation: A Step-By-Step Course on How to Meditate*
By Sharon Salzberg (2006)

*Wherever You Go, There You Are: Mindful Meditation in Everyday Life*
By Jon Kabat-Zinn (2009)

*Guided Mindfulness Meditation* (CD)
By: Jon Kabat-Zinn (2005)

*The Miracle of Mindfulness: An Introduction to the Practice of Meditation*
By Thich Nhat Hanh, Vo-Dinh Mai, and Mobi Ho (1999)

*How to Meditate: A Practical Guide*
By Kathleen McDonald and Robina Courtin (2005)
Recovery and Support Books and Resources

*Alcoholics Anonymous: The Big Book*
By Dr. Bob Smith and Bill Wilson (2011)

*The Twelve Steps and Twelve Traditions*
By Alcoholics Anonymous (2002)

*Alcoholics Anonymous: The Story of How Many Thousands of Men and Women Have Recovered from Alcoholism*
By Alcoholics Anonymous World Services (2002)

*Narcotics Anonymous*
By World Service Office (2008)

*It Works: How and Why: The Twelve Steps and Twelve Traditions of Narcotics Anonymous*
By World Service Office (1993)

*Narcotics Anonymous Step Working Guides*
By Narcotics Anonymous (2011)

*The Substance Abuse and Recovery Workbook*
By John J. Liptak and Ester Leutenberg, illustrated by Amy Brodsky (2008)
Educational Resources on Well-being
Know Yourself DVD Series
Anthropedia Foundation
www.anthropediafoundation.org

*Eating for Recovery: The Essential Nutrition Plan to Reverse the Physical Damage of Alcoholism*
By Molly Siple (2008)
USDA Food Guide Pyramid
Personal customization tool
www.choosemyplate.gov

*Recovery Health and Nutrition*
By Robert Jakobsen (2011)

*Lifestyle Changes: 12 Step Recovery and Diet Guide*
By Marilyn Rollins (1991)

*Recovery from Addiction*
By John Finnegan & Daphne Gray (1995)

*The New Pritikin Program*
By Robert Pritikin (2007)

*The Pritikin Edge: 10 Essential Ingredients for a Long and Delicious Life*
By Robert A. Vogel and Paul Tager Lehr (2010)

*The Anatomy of Addiction: Overcoming the Triggers that Stand in the Way of Recovery*
By Morteza Khaleghi and Karen Khaleghi (2011)

*12 Stupid Things that Mess Up Recovery: Avoiding Relapse through Self-Awareness and Right Action*
By: Allen Berger (2008)

*The Science of Spirituality: Integrating Science, Psychology, Philosophy, Spirituality, and Religion*
By Lee Bladon (2010)

*Healing the Addicted Brain: The Revolutionary, Science-based Alcoholism and Addiction Recovery Program*
By Harold Urschel (2009)

*Pocket Sponsor: 24/7 Back to the Basics Support for Addiction Recovery*
By Shelly Marshall (2003)

*The 10 Toughest Questions Families and Friends Ask about Addiction and Recovery*
DVD Starring Joe Herzanek (2010)

*Addict in the Family: Stories of Loss, Hope, and Recovery*
By Beverly Conyers (2003)

*Stage II Recovery: Life Beyond Addiction*
By Earnie Larsen (1984)

*Full Recovery: Creating a Personal Action Plan for Life Beyond Sobriety*
By Brian McAlister (2010)

*Overcoming Prescription Drug Addiction: A Guide to Coping and Understanding*
By Rod Cowin (2008)

*Tales of Addiction and Inspiration for Recovery: Twenty True Stories from the Soul*
By Barbara Sinor and Cardwell C. Nuckols (2010)

*First Year Sobriety: When All that Changes Is Everything*
By: Guy Kettelhack (1998)

*Out-of-Control: A Dialectical Behavior Therapy (DBT)–Cognitive Behavioral Therapy (CBT) Workbook for Getting Control of Our Emotions and Emotion-Driven Behavior*
By Melanie Gordon Sheets (2009)

*Creative Recovery: A Complete Addiction Treatment Program that Uses Your Natural Creativity*
By Eric Maisel and Susan Raeburn (2008)

*The Twelve Steps and Dual Disorders: A Framework of Recovery for Those of Us with Addiction and an Emotional or Psychiatric Illness*
By Pat Samples and Tim Hamilton (1994)

*Codependent No More: How to Stop Controlling Others and Start Caring for Yourself*
By Melody Beattie (1986)

*Codependent No More: Companion Workbook*
By Melody Beattie (2011)

*The Language of Letting Go*
By Melody Beattie (1990)

*Codependent No More: Beyond Codependency*
By Melody Beattie (2001)

*Codependents' Guide to the Twelve Steps*
By Melody Beattie (1992)

*Slaying the Dragon: The History of Addiction Treatment and Recovery in America*
By William L. White (1998)

*Addiction and Grace: Love and Spirituality in the Healing of Addictions (Plus)*
By Gerald G. May (2007)

*The Wisdom of Letting Go: The Path of the Wounded Soul*
By Leo Booth (2009)

*The Secret of Letting Go*
By Guy Finley (2002)
Books on Mindfulness

*Mindful Recovery: A Spiritual Path to Healing from Addiction*
By Thomas Bien and Beverly Bien (2002)

*Ordinary Recovery: Mindfulness, Addiction, and the Path of Lifelong Sobriety*
By William Alexander and Kevin Griffin (2010)

*The Mindfulness and Acceptance Workbook for Anxiety: A Guide to Breaking Free from Anxiety, Phobias, and Worry Using Acceptance and Commitment Therapy*
By John P. Forsyth and Georg H. Eifert (2008)

*The Mindfulness and Acceptance Workbook for Depression: Using Acceptance and Commitment Therapy to Move Through Depression and Create a Life Worth Living*
By Patricia Robinson and Kirk Strosahl (2008)

*Happiness: Essential Mindfulness Practices*
By Thich Nhat Nanh (2009)

**Positive Sobriety**

*Real Happiness: The Power of Meditation: A 28-Day Program*
By Sharon Salzberg

*Savor: Mindful Eating, Mindful Life*
By Thich Nhat Hanh and Lilian Cheung (2011)

*The Zen of Eating*
By Ronna Kabatznick (1998)

*How to Train a Wild Elephant: And Other Adventures in Mindfulness*
By Jan Chozen Bays (2011)

*Mindfulness in Plain English*
By Bhante Henepola Gunaratana (1996)
Books on Happiness

*Happier: Learn the Secrets to Daily Joy and Lasting Fulfillment*
By Tal Ben-Shahar (2007)

*Even Happier: A Gratitude Journal of Daily Joy and Lasting Fulfillment*
By Tal Ben-Shahar (2009)

*The Question of Happiness: On Finding Meaning, Pleasure, and the Ultimate Currency*
By Tal Ben-Shahar (2002)

*Happiness: A Guide to Developing Life's Most Important Skill*
By Matthieu Ricard and Daniel Goleman (2007)

*Twelve Steps to Happiness*
By Joe Klass, Jennifer Schneider, Gayle Rossellini, and Mark Worden (1990)

*Higher and Higher: From Drugs and Destruction to Health and Happiness*
By Jost Sauer (2007)

*Steps to Happiness: Travelling from Depression and Addiction to the Buddhist Path*
By Taranatha (2006)

*Spiritual Engineering: The New Science for Happiness and Extraordinary Relationships*
By Thomas Strawser, Mary Anne Maier and Patricia Strawser (2010)

*Think Right, Feel Right: The Building Block for Happiness and Emotional Well-being*
By Robert Isett and Brian Isett (2010)

*Choosing Happiness: The Art of Living Unconditionally*
By Veronica Ray (1991)

*Conquering Addiction: A Guide for Maintaining Happiness Regardless of Circumstance*
By J. J. Goldway (2011)

*Addicted to Unhappiness: Free Yourself from the Moods and Behaviors that Undermine Relationships, Work, and the Life You Want*
By Martha Pieper and William Pieper (2004)

*When Misery Is Company: End Self-Sabotage and Become Content*
By Anne Katherine (2004)

*The Happiness Trap: How to Stop Struggling and Start Living*
By Russ Harris and Steven Hayes (2008)

*The Happiness Hypothesis: Finding Modern Truth in Ancient Wisdom*
By Jonathan Haidt (2006)

*The Art of Happiness, 10th Anniversary Edition: A Handbook for Living*
By The Dalai Lama (2009)

*The How of Happiness: A New Approach to Getting the Life You Want*
By Sonja Lyubomirsky (2008)

*Authentic Happiness: Using the New Positive Psychology to Realize Your Potential for Lasting Fulfillment*
By Martin E. P. Seligman (2003)

*Happiness: Unlocking the Mysteries of Psychological Wealth*
By Ed Diener and Robert Biswas-Diener (2008)

*Happiness*
By Joan Chittister (2011)

*Buddha's Brain: The Practical Neuroscience of Happiness, Love, and Wisdom*
By Rick Hanson and Richard Mendius (2009)

**Positive Sobriety**

*The Joy of Living: Unlocking the Secret and Science of Happiness*
By Yongley Mingyur Rinpoche, Eric Swanson and Daniel Goleman (2008)

*Flourish: A Visionary New Understanding of Happiness and Well-being*
By Martin E. P. Seligman (2011)

# References

Akisal, K., M. Savino, H. Akisal. 2005. Temperament profiles in physicians, lawyers, managers, industrialists, architects, journalists, and artists: A study in psychiatric outpatients. *Journal of Affective Disorders* 85:201–206.

Alcoholics Anonymous. 1953. *Twelve Steps and Twelve Traditions*. New York: Alcoholics Anonymous World Services.

———. 1976. *Alcoholics Anonymous*, 3rd edition. New York: Alcoholics Anonymous World Services.

———. 1990. *Alcoholics Anonymous*. New York: Alcoholics Anonymous World Services.

Alexander, W. 1997. *Cool water: Alcoholism, mindfulness, and ordinary recovery*. Boston: Shambhala Publications.

Allport, G. 1937. *Personality: A psychological interpretation*. New York: Holt, Rinehart & Winston.

Amen, D. G. 1998. *Change your brain, change your life: The breakthrough program for conquering anxiety, depression, obsessiveness, anger, and impulsiveness*. New York: Three Rivers Press.

*American Heritage Dictionary of the English Language*. 2000. Boston: Houghton-Mifflin.

American Medical Association (AMA). 1956. AMA history: 1941–1960. Retrieved from http://ama-assn.org.

American Psychiatric Association. 2000. Diagnostic and statistical manual of mental disorders, 4th edition, text revision. Washington, D.C.: American Psychiatric Publishing.

American Society of Addiction Medicine. 2006. *Expanding treatment of opioid dependence: Initial physician and patient experiences with the adoption of buprenorphine.* U.S. Department of Health and Human Services. SAMHSA. http://buprenorphine.samhsa.gov/ASAM_06_Final_Results.pdf.

American Society of Addiction Medicine. 2011. *Public policy statement: Definition of addiction,* August 15. Accessed September 29, 2011, from www.asam.org/1defininion_of_addicion_long_4-11.pdf.

Anderson, D. 1981. *Perspectives in treatment: The Minnesota experience.* Center City, MN: Hazelden Educational Service.

Angevaren, M., G. Aufdemkampe, H. J. Verhaar, A. Aleman, L. Vanhees. 2008. Physical activity and enhanced fitness improve cognitive function in older people without known cognitive impairment. *Cochrane Database Systematic Review* 2 (April 16): CD005381.

Angres, D. H. 2010. The Temperament and Character Inventory in addiction treatment. *Focus: The Journal of Lifelong Learning in Psychiatry* 8 (2): 187–197.

Angres, D. H., K. Bettinardi-Angres. 2008. The disease of addiction: Origins, treatment, and Recovery. *Disease-A-Month* 54(10): 691–722.

Angres, D. H., M. P. McGovern, M. F. Shaw, P. Rawal. 2003. Psychiatric comorbidity and physicians with substance use disorders: A comparison between the 1980s and 1990s. *Journal of Addictive Disease* 22:79–87.

Angres, D. H., G. D. Talbott, K. Bettinardi-Angres. 1998. *Healing the healer: The addicted physician.* Madison, CT: Psychosocial Press.

Angres, D., A. Nielsen. 2007. The role of the TCI (Temperament and Character Inventory) in individualized treatment planning in a population of addicted professionals. *Journal of Addictive Disease* 26:51–64.

Anonymous. 1999. *Co-Dependents Anonymous,* Phoenix, AZ: Co-Dependents Anonymous.

Arnau, M. M., S. Mondon, J. J. Santacreu. 2008. Using the Temperament and Character Inventory (TCI) to predict outcome after inpatient detoxification during 100 days of outpatient treatment. *Alcohol and Alcoholism* 43:583–588.

Ash, M. 1993. *The Zen of recovery.* New York: The Putman Publishing Group.

# References

Bahrke, M., and W. Morgan. 1978. Anxiety reduction following exercise and meditation. *Cognitive Therapy and Research* 2:323–333.

Baker, D., C. Greenberg, I. L. Yalof. 2008. *What happy women know: How new findings in positive psychology can change women's lives for the better.* New York: St. Martin's Griffin.

Baldisseri, M. R. 2007. Impaired healthcare professional. *Critical Care Medicine* 35 (2): s106–s116.

Ball, S. A., H. Tennen, J. C. Poling, H. R. Kranzler, B. J. Rounsaville. 1997. Personality, temperament, and character dimensions and the DSM-IV personality disorders in substance abusers. *Journal of Abnormal Psychology* 106 (4): 545–553.

Basiaux, P., O. le Bon, M. Dramaix, I. Massat, D. Souery, J. Mendlewicz, I. Pelc, P. Verbank. 2001. Temperament and Character Inventory (TCI) personality profile and sub-typing in alcoholic patients: A controlled study. *Alcohol and Alcoholism* 36 (6): 584–587.

Battaglia, M., T. R. Przybeck, L. Bellodi, C. R. Cloninger. 1996. Temperament dimensions explain the comorbidity of psychiatric disorders. *Comprehensive Psychiatry* 37 (4): 292–298.

Bayon, C., K. Hill, D. M. Svrakic, T. R. Przybeck, C. R. Cloninger. 1996. Dimensional assessment of personality in an outpatient sample: Relations of the systems of Millon and Cloninger. *Journal of Psychiatric Research* 30 (5): 341–352.

Beattie, M. 1986. *Codependent no more: How to stop controlling others and start caring for yourself.* Center City, MN: Hazelden Publications.

Beck, A. T., A. J. Rush, B. F. Shaw, G. Emery. 1979. *Cognitive therapy of depression.* New York: The Guilford Press.

Beck, A. T., F. Wright, C. Newman, B. Liesi. 1993. *Cognitive therapy of substance abuse.* New

Belcher, Annabelle, Volkow, F Nora. Moeller, Gerard and Ferre, Sergi 2104. *Personality traits and vulnerability or resilience to substance use disorders* The Guilford Press.

Ben-Shahar, T. 2007. *Happier: Learn the secrets to daily joy and lasting fulfillment.* New York: McGraw-Hill.

———. 2009. *The pursuit of perfect: How to stop chasing perfection and start living a richer, happier life.* New York: McGraw-Hill.

Benson, H. and R. K. Wallace. 1972. Decreased drug abuse with Transcendental Meditation: A study of 1,862 subjects. In *Drug abuse: Proceedings of the international conference*, edited by C. J. D. Zarafonetis, 369–376. Philadelphia: Lea and Febiger.

Berge, K. H., M. D. Seppala, A. M. Schipper. 2009. Chemical dependency and the physician. *Mayo Clinical Proceedings* 84 (7): 625–631.

Berridge, K. C., and M. L. Kringelbach. 2008. Affective neuroscience of pleasure: Rewards in humans and other animals. *Psychopharmacology* 199:457–480.

Bettinardi-Angres, K., and D. Angres. 2010. Understanding the disease of addiction. *Journal of Nursing Regulation* 1 (2): 31–37.

Biswas-Diener, R., and B. Dean. 2007. *Positive psychology coaching: Putting the science of happiness to work for your clients.* Hoboken, NJ: John Wiley & Sons.

Blum, K., J. G. Cull, E. R. Braverman, D. E. Comings. 1996. Reward deficiency syndrome: Addictive impulse and compulsive disorders may have a common genetic basis. *American Scientist* 84(2): 132.

Blumenthal, J. A., M. A. Babyak, K. A. Moore, W. E. Craighead, S. Herman, P. Khatri R. Waugh, , et al. 1999. Effects of exercise training on older patients with major depression. *Archives of Internal Medicine* 159:2349–2356.

Blumenthal, J.A., R. Sanders Williams, T. L. Needels, A. G. Wallace. 1982. Psychological changes accompany aerobic exercise in healthy middle-aged adults. *Psychosomatic Medicine* 44 (6): 529–536.

Bohigan, G. M., R. Bondurant, J. Croughan. 2005. The impaired and disruptive physician: The Missouri physician's health program: An update. *Journal of Addictive Disease* 24:13–23.

Bohman, M., C. R. Cloninger, S. Sigvardsson, A. L. von Knorring. 1987. The genetics of alcoholisms and related disorders. *Journal of Psychiatric Research* 24 (4): 447–452.

Bolte-Taylor, J. 2008. *My stroke of insight: A brain scientist's personal journey.* New York: Viking Penguin.

Boly, M., C. Phillips, L. Tshibanda, A. Vanhaudenhuyse, M. Schabus, T. T. Dang-Vu, G. Moonen, R. Hustinx, P. Maquet, S. Laureys. 2008. Intrinsic brain activity in altered states of consciousness: How conscious is the default mode of brain function? *Annals of the New York Academy of Science* 1129:119–129.

Bond, J., L. Kaskutas, C. Weisner. 2003. The persistent influence of social networks and Alcoholics Anonymous on abstinence. *Journal of Studies on Alcohol* 64:579–588.

Boren, J. J., K. Carroll, National Institute on Drug Abuse. 2000. Approaches to drug abuse counseling. Bethesda, MD: National Institute on Drug Abuse, Division of Treatment and Research Development, Behavioral Treatment Development Branch.

Bowen, S., N. Chawla, S. E. Collins, K. Witkiewitz, S. Hsu, J. Grow, S. Clifasefi, M. et al. 2009. Mindfulness-based stress relapse prevention for substance use disorders: A pilot efficacy trial. *Substance Abuse* 30: 295–305. .

Bradshaw, J. 2005. *Healing the shame that binds you*. Deerfield Beach, FL: Health Communications (Orig. pub. 1988.)

Brickman, P., and D. T. Campbell. 1971. Hedonic relativism and the good society. In *Adaptation Level Theory: A Symposium*, edited by M. H. Appley, 287–302. New York: Academic Press.

Brogaard, B. 2010. Anger and aggressive behavior. Livestrong, July 10. www.livestrong.com/article/170803-anger-aggressive-behavior/

Brown, R. A., A. M. Abrantes, J. P. Read, B. H. Marcus, J. Jakicic, D. R. Strong, J. R. Oakley, S. E. Ramsey, C. W. Kahler, G. G. Stuart, M. E. Dubreuil, A. A. Gordon. 2010. A pilot study of aerobic exercise as an adjunctive treatment for drug dependence. *Mental Health and Physical Activity* 3 (1): 27–34.

Brown, R. P., and P. L. Gerbarg. 2005. Sudarshan kriya yogic breathing in the treatment of stress, anxiety, and depression: Part ii—Clinical applications and guidelines. *Journal of Alternative and Complementary Medicine*, 11:711–717.

Buchowski, M. S., N. N. Meade, E. Charboneau, S. Park, M. S. Dietrich, R. L. Cowan, P. R. Martin. 2011. Aerobic exercise training reduces cannabis craving and use in non-treatment seeking cannabis-dependent adults. *PLoS ONE* 6(3): e17465. doi: 10.1371/journal.pone.0017465.

Bouchard, Thomas J.; McGue, Matt (2003). "Genetic and environmental influences on human psychological differences". *Journal of Neurobiology*

Burney, R. 1995. *Codependence: The dance of wounded souls*. Cambria, CA: Joy to You and Me Enterprises.

Burns, D. 1999. *Feeling good, revised edition*. New York: Avon Books.

Byrne, A., and D. G. Byrne. 1993. The effects of exercise on depression, anxiety, and other mood states: A review. *Journal of Psychosomatic Research* 37 (6): 565–574.

Carnes, P. 1993. *A gentle path through the twelve steps: The classic guide for all people in the process of recovery*. Center City, MN: Hazelden Publishing.

———. 2004. Handbook of addictive disorders: A practical guide to diagnosis and treatment. Edited by Coombs, R. H. Hoboken, NJ: John Wiley & Sons, s.v. "addiction interaction disorder."

Carpentier, P. J., C. A. De Jong, B. A. G. Dijkstra, C. A. G. Verbrugge, P. F. M. Krabbe. 2005. A controlled trial of methylphenidate in adults with attention deficit/hyperactivity disorder and substance use disorders. *Addiction* 100 (12): 1868–1874.

Carroll, K. 2000. *A cognitive behavioral approach: Treating cocaine addiction*. Rockville, MD: National Institute of Drug Addiction.

Center for Substance Abuse Treatment. 2005. Substance abuse treatment: Group therapy. Treatment Improvement Protocol (TIP) series 41. DHHS Publication No. (SMA) 05-3991. Rockville, MD: Substance Abuse and Mental Health Services Administration.

Centers for Disease Control and Prevention. 2008. Smoking-attributable mortality, years of potential life lost, and productivity losses: United States, 2000–2004. *Morbidity and Mortality Weekly Report* 57 (45): 1226–1228.

Chakroun, N., E. I. Johnson, J. Swendsen. 2010. Mood and personality-based models of substance use. *Psychology of Addictive Behaviors* 24 (1), 129–136.

Chodron, P. 1997. *When things fall apart: Heart advice for difficult times*. Boston: Shambhala Publications.

Clark, L. A. 1990. Toward a consensual set of symptom clusters for assessment of personality disorder. In *Advances in personality disorder*, edited by N. Butcher and C. D. Spielberger, 243–266. Hillsdale, NJ: Erlbaum.

Cloninger, C. R. 1987. A systematic method for clinical description and classification of personality variants. *Archives of General Psychiatry* 44:573–588.

———. 1987. Neurogenic adaptive mechanisms in alcoholism. *Science* 236:410–416.

———. 1987. Recent advances in family studies of alcoholism. *Progress in clinical and biological research* 241:47–60.

———. (1994). Temperament and personality. *Current Opinion in Neurobiology* 4 (2): 266–273.

———. 1997. A 15 step model of personality development: Assessment and treatment implications for alcoholism. In *The long and the short of treatment for alcohol and drug disorders*, edited by J. D. Sellman, G. M. Robinson, R. McCormick, G. M. Dore, 45–76. Christchurch, NZ: Department of Psychological Medicine, Christchurch School of Medicine.

———, ed. 1999. Personality and psychopathology. American Psychopathological Association Series. Washington, D.C.: American Psychiatric Press.

———. 2000. Biology of personality dimensions. *Current Opinion in Psychiatry* 13 (6): 611–616.

———. 2004. Feeling good: The science of well-being. New York: Oxford University Press.

———. 2006. The science of well-being: an integrated approach to mental health and its disorders. *World Psychiatry* 5:71–76.

———. 2007. Spirituality and the science of feeling good. *Southern Medical Journal* 100 (7): 740–743.

———. 2011. *TCI-R US norms tables*. Unpublished manuscript.

———. 2006 The science of well-being: An integrated approach to mental health and its disorders. *World Psychiatry*, 5 (2): 71–76.

Cloninger, C. R., and A. H. Zohar. 2011. Personality and the perception of health and happiness. *Journal of Affective Disorders* 128 (1-2): 24–32.

Cloninger, C. R., A. H. Zohar, S. Hirschmann, D. Dahan. 2012. The psychological costs and benefits of being highly persistent: Personality profiles distinguish mood disorders from anxiety disorders. *Journal of Affective Disorders*, 136 (3): 758–766.

Cloninger, C. R., D. M. Svrakic, T. R. Przybeck. 1993. A psychobiological model of temperament and character. *Archives of General Psychiatry* 50:975–990.

Cloninger, C. R., T. R. Przybeck, D. M. Svrakic, R. D. Wetzel. 1994. The Temperament and Character Inventory (TCI): A guide to its development and use. St Louis, MO: Center for Psychobiology of Personality, Washington University.

Colcombe, S., and A. F. Kramer. 2003. Fitness effects on the cognitive function of older adults: A meta-analytic study. *Psychological Science* 14 (2): 125–130.

Cole, B., and K. I. Pargament. 1999. Spiritual surrender: A paradoxical path to control. In *Integrating spirituality into treatment: Resources for practitioners.* Edited by W. Miller, 179–198. Washington, D.C.: APA Press.

Compton, W. C. 2005. An introduction to positive psychology. Australia; Belmont, CA: Thompson/Wadsworth.

Compton, W. M., and N. D. Volkow. 2006. Abuse of prescription drugs and the risk of addiction. *Drug and Alcohol Dependence* 83 (1): S4–S7.

Compton. W. M., Y. F. Thomas, F. S. Stinson, B. F. Grant. 2007. Prevalence, correlates, disability, and comorbidity of *DSM-IV* drug abuse and dependence in the United States: Results from the National Epidemiologic Survey on Alcohol and Related Conditions. *Archives of General Psychiatry* 64:566–576.

Consumer Reports. 1995. Mental health: Does therapy help? (November): 734–739.

Costa, P. T., and R. R. McCrae. 1989. *The NEO-PI/NEO-FFI manual supplement.* Odessa, FL: Psychological Assessment Resources, Inc.

Csikszentmihalyi, M. 1990. *Flow: The psychology of optimal experience.* New York: Harper Perennial.

Csikszentmihalyi, M., and I. S. Csikszentmihalyi. 2006. *A life worth living: Contributions to positive psychology.* New York: Oxford University Press.

Dagher, A., and T. W. Robbins. 2009. Personality, addiction, dopamine: Insights from Parkinson's disease. *Neuron* 61 (4): 502-510.

Davidson, R. J., J. Kabat-Zinn, J. Schumacher, M. Rosenkranz, D. Muller, S. F. Santorelli, F. Urbanowski, A. Harrington, K. Bonus, J. F. Sheridan. 2003. Alterations in brain and immune function produced by mindfulness meditation. *Psychosomatic Medicine* 65 (4): 564–570.

Davis, L. 1990. *The courage to heal workbook.* New York: Harper Perennial.

De Leon, G. 2000. *The therapeutic community: Theory, model, and method.* New York: Springer Publishing Company.

De Moja, C. A. 1997. Scores on locus of control and aggression for drug addicts, users, and controls. *Psychological Reports* 80:40–42.

# References

De Moja, C. A., and C. D. Spielberger. 1997. Anger and drug addiction. *Psychological Reports* 81:152–154.

Descartes, R. 1641. Meditations on first philosophy. In *The philosophical writings of René Descartes*, vol. 2. Translated by J. Cottingham, R. Stoothoff, and D. Murdoch, 1–62. Cambridge: Cambridge University Press, 1984.

Devor, E. J., and C. R. Cloninger. 1989. Genetics of alcoholism. *Annual Review of Genetics* 23:19–36.

Dick, D. M., and L. J. Beirut. 2006. The genetics of alcohol dependence. *Current Psychiatry Reports*. 8:151–157.

DiClemente, C. C. 2006. *Addiction and change: How addictions develop and addicted people recover*. New York: Guilford Press.

Diener, E., and R. Biswas-Diener. 2008. *Happiness: Unlocking the secrets of psychological wealth*. Malden, MA: Blackwell Publishing.

Diener, E., R. E. Lucas, C. N. Scollon. 2006. Beyond the hedonic treadmill: Revising the adaptation theory of well-being. *American Psychologist* 61 (4): 305-314.

Dodrill, C. L., D. A. Helmer, T. R. Kosten. 2011. Prescription pain management dependence. *American Journal of Psychiatry* 168 (5): 466–471.

Donnellan, M.B., Oswald, F.L., Baird, B.M., & Lucas, R.E. (2006). The mini-IPIP scales: Tiny-yet-effective measures of the Big Five factors of personality. *Psychological Assessment, 18*, 192-203.

Domino, K. B., T. F. Hornbein, N. L. Polissar, G. Renner, J. Johnson, S. Alberti, L. Hankes. 2005. Risk factors for relapse in health care professionals with substance use disorders. *Journal of the American Medical Association* 293 (12): 1453–1460.

Dowd, M. (2008). *Thank God for evolution: How the marriage of science and religion will transform your life and our world*. New York: Viking Penguin.

Dunn, A. L., M. H. Trivedi, J. B. Kampert, C. G. Clark, H. O. Chambliss. 2005. Exercise treatment for depression: Efficacy and dose response. *American Journal of Preventive Medicine* 28 (1): 1–8.

DuPont, R. L., A. T. McLellan, W. L. White, L. J. Merlo, M. S. Gold. 2009. Setting the standard for recovery: Physicians' Health Programs. *Journal of Substance Abuse Treatment* 36 (2): 159–171.

Dyer, W. W. 2004. *The power of intention: Learning to co-create your world your way*. CA: Hay House, Inc.

Edenberg, H. J. 2003. The collaborative study on the genetics of alcoholism: An update. National Institute on Alcohol Abuse and Alcoholism (NIAAA). Accessed September 29, 2011, http://pubs.niaaa.nih.gov/publications/arh26-3/214-218.htm.

Egendorf, A. 1995. Hearing people through their pain. *Journal of Traumatic Stress* 8:5–28.

Ellis, A., and I. Becker. 1986. A guide to personal happiness. North Hollywood, CA: Wilshire Book Company.

Emmons, R. 2007. *Thanks! How the new science of gratitude can make you happier.* New York: Houghton Mifflin.

Erickson, K. I., M. W. Voss, R. S. Prakash, C. Basak, A. Szabo, L. Chaddock, J. S. Kim, et al.. 2011. Exercise training increases size of hippocampus and improves memory. *Proceedings of the National Academy of Sciences of the United States of America*, 108 (7): 3017–3022. www.pnas.org/cgi/doi/10.1073/pnas.1015950108.

Etnier, J. L., P. M. Nowell, D. M. Landers, B. A. Sibley. 2006. A meta-regression to examine the relationship between aerobic fitness and cognitive performance. *Brain Research Reviews* 52:119–130.

Farmer, R. F., and L. R. Goldberg. 2008. Brain modules, personality layers, planes of being, spiral structures, and the equally implausible distinction between TCI-R "temperament and character" scales: Reply to Cloninger, *Psychological Assessment* 20 (3): 300–304.

Fehmi, L., and J. Robbins. 2007. The Open-Focus brain: Harnessing the power of attention to heal mind and body. Boston: Trumpeter.

Fernandez-Montalvo, J., N. Landa, J. M. Lopez-Goni, I. Lorea. 2006. Personality disorders in alcoholics: A comparative pilot study between the IPDE and the MCMI-II. *Addictive Behaviors* 31:1442–1448.

Firestone, R. W. 1987. The fantasy bond: Structure of psychological defenses. Santa Barbara, CA: The Glendon Association.

Forsyth, J. P., and G. H. Eifert. 2007. The mindfulness and acceptance workbook for anxiety: A guide to breaking free from anxiety, phobias, and worry using acceptance and commitment therapy. Oakland, CA: New Harbinger Publications, Inc.

Frankl, V. 1959. Man's search for meaning. Boston: Beacon Press.

# References

Fregni, F., P. S. Boggio, M. A. Nitsche, S. P. Rigonatti, A. Pascual-Leone. 2006. Cognitive effects of repeated sessions of transcranial direct current stimulation in patients with depression. *Depression and Anxiety* 23:482–484.

Freud, S. 1960. Civilization and its discontents. New York: W. W. Norton & Company.

Galanter, M. et.al. (2011). Introducing Spirituality into Psychiatric Care; J. of Relig. Health, 50:81-91.

Galin, D. 2001. The concept "self" and "person" in Buddhism and in Western psychology. In *Meeting at the roots: Essays on Tibetan Buddhism and the natural sciences*, edited by B. Alan Wallace. New York: Columbia University Press.

Gallegos, K. V., B. H. Lubin, C. Bowers, J. W. Blevins, G. D. Talbott, P. O. Wilson. (1992). Relapse and recovery: Five to ten year follow-up study of chemically dependent physicians—the Georgia experience. *Maryland Medical Journal* 41:315–319.

Gaskell, K. J. 2010. Anger and alcoholism. Livestrong, March 23. www.livestrong.com/article/85504-anger-alcoholism/.

George, S. M., J. P. Connor, M. J. Gullo, R. Young McD. 2010. A prospective study of personality features predictive of early adolescent alcohol misuse. *Personality and Individual Differences* 49:204–209.

Gianoulakis, C., B. Krishnan, J. Thavundayil. 1996. Enhanced sensitivity of pituitary beta-endorphin to ethanol in subjects at high risk of alcoholism. *Archives of General Psychiatry* 53 (3):250–257.

Gillespie, N. A., C. R. Cloninger, A. C. Heath, N. G. Martin. 2003. The genetic and environmental relationship between Cloninger's dimensions of temperament and character. *Personality and Individual Differences* 35 (8): 1931–1946.

Glass, I. B. 1991. *The international handbook of addiction behavior.* New York; London: Tavistock/Routledge.

Goldman, D., G. Oroszi, F. Ducci. 2005. The genetics of addictions: Uncovering the genes. *National Review of Genetics* 6:521–532. Laboratory, Air Force Systems Command, 1961

Goldberg, L. R. (1993). "The structure of phenotypic personality traits". *American Psychologist*

Goldberg, L. R., Johnson, J. A., Eber, H. W., Hogan, R., Ashton, M. C., Cloninger, C. R., & Gough, H. C. (2006). The International Personality Item Pool and the future of public-domain personality measures. Journal of Research in Personality, 40, 84-96.

Goldstein, R. Z., N. D. Volkow. 2002. Drug addiction and its underlying neurobiological basis: Neuroimaging evidence for the involvement of the frontal cortex. *The American Journal of Psychiatry* 159 (10): 1642–1652.

Goleman, D., Dalai Lama. 2003. *Destructive emotions: How can we overcome them: A scientific dialogue with the Dalai Lama*. New York: Bantam Dell.

Gorenstein, E. E. 1984. Debating mental illness: Implications for science, medicine, and social policy. *American Psychologist* 39 (1): 50–56.

Graham, T., and D. Ramsey. 2011. *The happiness diet: A nutritional prescription for a sharp brain, balanced mood, and lean, energized body*. New York: Rodale Books.

Grant, B. F., F. S. Stinson, D. A. Dawson, S. P. Chou, M.C. Dufour, W. Compton, R. P. Pickering, K. Kaplan. 2004. Co-occurrence of 12-month alcohol and drug use disorders and personality disorders in the United States. *Archives of General Psychiatry* 61:361–368.

Grekin, E. R., K. J. Sher, P. K. Wood. 2006. Personality and substance dependence symptoms: Modeling substance-specific traits. *Psychology of Addictive Behaviors* 20:415–424.

Grucza, R. A., C. R. Cloninger, K. K. Bucholz, J. N. Constantino, M. I. Schuckit, D. M. Dick, L. J. Bierut. 2006. Novelty seeking as a moderator of familial risk for alcohol dependence. *Alcoholism: Clinical and Experimental Research* 30 (7): 1176–1183.

Gulliver, S. B., B. W. Kamholz, A. W. Helstrom. 2006. Smoking cessation and alcohol abstinence: What do the data tell us? *Alcohol Research and Health* 29 (3): 208–212.

Gunaratana, B. H. 2002. *Mindfulness in plain English*. Boston, MA: Wisdom Publications.

Guze, S. B., C. R. Cloninger, R. Martin, P. J. Clayton. 1986. Alcoholism as a medical disorder. *Comprehensive Psychiatry* 27 (6): 501–510.

Harkness, A. R., J. L. McNulty. 1994. The personality psychopathology five (PSY-5): Issue from the pages of a diagnostic manual instead of a dictionary. In *Differentiating Normal and Abnormal Personality*, edited by S. Strack and M. Lorr, 291–315. New York: Springer.

Hasin, D. S., F. S. Stinson, E. Ogburn, B. F. Grant. 2007. Prevalence, correlates, disability, and comorbidity of DSM-IV alcohol abuse and dependence in the United States. *Archives of General Psychiatry* 64 (7): 830–842.

Hattori, S., M. Naoi, H. Nishino. 1994. Striatal dopamine turnover during treadmill running in the rat: Relation to the speed of running. *Brain Research Bulletin*, 35 (1): 41–49.

Hayes, S. C. K. D. Strosahl, K. G. Wilson. 1999. *Acceptance and Commitment Therapy: An experiential approach to behavior change*. New York: Guilford Press.

Hayes, S. C., K. G. Wilson, E. Gifford, R. Bissett, M. Piasecki, S. Batten, M. Byrd, J. Gregg. 2004. A preliminary trial of twelve-step facilitation and acceptance and commitment therapy with polysubstance-abusing methadone-maintained opiate addicts. *Behavior Therapy*, 35: 667-688.

Heilig, M., D. Goldman, W. Berrettini, C. P. O'Brien. 2011. Pharmacogenetic approaches to the treatment of alcohol addiction. *Nature Reviews Neuroscience*, 12: 670-684.

Heinz, A., T. Siessmeier, J. Wrase, H. G. Bucholv, G. Grunder, Y. Kumakura, P. Cumming, M. Schreckenberger, M. N. Smolka, F. Rosch, K. Mann, P. Bartenstein. 2004. Correlation of alcohol craving with striatal dopamine synthesis capacity and d2/3 receptor availability: A combined (18F) dopa and (18F) DMFP PET study in detoxified alcoholic patients. *The American Journal of Psychiatry* 162:1515–1520.

Heisenberg, W. 1930. *The physical principles of the quantum theory*. Chicago: University of Chicago Press.

Heit, H. A., and D. L. Gourlay. 2008. Buprenorphine: New tricks with an old molecule for pain management. *Clinical Journal of Pain* 24 (2): 93–97.

Hesse, M., P. Nielsen, R. Rojskjaelr. 2007. Stability and change in Millon Clinical Multiaxial Inventory II personality disorder scores in treated alcohol dependent subjects: Relationship to post-treatment abstinence. *International Journal of Mental Health Addiction* 5:254–262.

Heyn, P., B. C. Abreu, K. J. Ottenbacher. 2004. The effects of exercise training on elderly persons with cognitive impairment and dementia: A meta-analysis. *Archives of Phyical Medicine and Rehabilitation*, 85 (10): 1694–1704.

Higgins, E. S., and M. S. George. 2009. *Brain stimulation therapies for clinicians*. Washington, D.C.: American Psychiatric Publishing, Inc.

Hoffman, N. G., and N. S. Miller. 1992. Treatment outcomes for abstinence-based programs. *Psychiatric Annals* 22 (8): 402–408.

Hoffmann, N. G., P. A. Harrison, C. A. Belille. 1983. Alcoholics Anonymous after treatment: Attendance and abstinence. *International Journal of the Addictions* 18 (3): 311–318.

Hoffmann, N. G., and R. A. Kaplan. 1991. *CATOR report: One year outcome for adolescents—key correlates and benefits of recovery.* St. Paul, MN: CATOR/New Standards, Inc.

Hogan, R., J. Johnson, S. R. Briggs. 1997. *Handbook of personality psychology.* San Diego, CA: Academic Press.

Howard, K. I., K. Moras, P. L. Brill, Z. Martinovich, W. Lutz. 1996. Evaluation of psychotherapy: Efficacy, effectiveness, and patient progress. *American Psychologist* 51: 1059–1064.

Hubbard, R. I. 1997. Overview of 1 year follow-up in the drug abuse treatment outcome study (DATOS). *Psychology of Addictive Behaviors* 11:264–278.

Huebner, H. F. 1993. *Endorphins, eating disorders, and other addictive behaviors.* New York: Norton.

Hughes, C. M. 2001. *Substance abuse and the nation's number one health problem.* Princeton, NJ: Robert Wood Johnson Foundation.

Hughes, P. H., N. Brandenburg, D. C. Baldwin, Jr., C. L. Storr, J. C. Anthony, D. V. Sheehan. 1992. Prevalence of substance use among U.S. physicians, *Journal of the American Medical Association* 267 (17): 2333–2339. Published correction appears in *Journal of the American Medical Association.* 1992. 268 (18): 2518.

Humphreys, K., and R. Moos. 2001. Can encouraging substance abuse patients to participate in self-help groups reduce demand for health care? *Alcoholism* 5 (25): 711–716.

Hyman, S. E. 2005. Addiction: A disease of learning and memory. *American Journal of Psychiatry* 162:1414–1422.

Insel, T. R. 2003. Is social attachment an addictive disorder? *Physiological Behavior* 79: 351–357.

Institute of Medicine. 2006. *Improving the quality of health care for mental and substance-use conditions.* Washington, D. C.: The National Academies Press.

James, W. 1997. The varieties of religious experience. New York: Simon & Schuster.

Jellinek, E. M. 1960. *The disease concept of alcoholism.* New Haven, CT: Yale Center for Alcoholic Studies.

Johnson, Paul M., Paul J. Kenny. 2010. Dopamine D2 receptors in addiction-like reward dysfunction and compulsive eating in obese rats. *Nature Neuroscience,* 13 (5): 635–641.

# References

Joseffson, K., C. R. Cloninger, M. Hintsanen, M. Jokela, L. Pulkki-Raback, L. Keltikangas-Jarvinen. 2011. Associations of personality profiles with various aspects of well-being: A population-based study. *Journal of Affective Disorders* 133 (1–2): 265–273.

Kabat-Zinn, J. 1990. *Full catastrophe living: Using the wisdom of your body and mind to face stress, pain, and illness.* New York: Dell Publishing.

———. 1994. *Wherever you go, there you are: Mindfulness meditation in everyday life.* New York: Hyperion.

———. 2005. *Coming to our senses: Healing ourselves and the world through mindfulness.* New York: Hyperion.

Kahneman, D., E. Diener, N. Schwartz, editors. 2003. *Well-being: The foundations of hedonic psychology.* New York: Russell Sage Foundation Publications.

Kalivas, P. W. 2003. Predisposition to addiction: Pharmacokinetics, pharmacodynamics, and brain circuitry. *The American Journal of Psychiatry* 160 (1): 1–3.

Kalivas, P. W., N. D. Volkow. 2005. The neural basis of addiction: A pathology of motivation and choice. *American Journal of Psychiatry* 162:1403–1413.

Kaplan, G., and R. Hammer, editors. 2002. *Brain circuitry and signaling in psychiatry.* Washington, D.C.: American Psychiatric Publishing.

Kaskutas, L. A. 2005. Alcoholics Anonymous careers: Patterns of AA involvement five years after treatment entry. *Alcohol Clinical and Experimental Research* 29:1983–1990.

Kaskutas, L. A., J. Bond, K. Humphreys. 2002. Social networks as mediators of the effect of Alcoholics Anonymous. *Addiction* 97:891–900.

Kaskutas, L. A., M. S. Subbaraman, J. Witbrodt, S. E. Zemore. 2009. Effectiveness of making Alcoholics Anonymous easier. A group format 12-step facilitation approach. *Journal of Substance Abuse Treatment* 37:228–239.

Kauer, J. A., and R. C. Malenka. 2007. Synaptic plasticity and addiction. *Nature Reviews Neuroscience* 8 (11): 844–858.

Kaufman, M., editor. 2001. *Brain imaging in substance abuse.* Totowa, NJ: Humana Press.

Kelly, J. F., J. McKellar, R. Moos. 2003. Major depression in patients with substance use disorders: Relationship to 12-step self-help involvement and substance use outcomes. *Addiction* 4 (98): 499–508.

Keltner, D. 2009. *Born to be good: The science of a meaningful life*. New York: W. W. Norton & Company.

Kenna, G. A., and M. D. Wood. 2005. The prevalence of alcohol, cigarette, and illicit drug use and problems among dentists. *Journal of the American Dental Association* 136:1023–1032.

Keyes, C. L., D. Shmotkin, C. D. Ryff. 2002. Optimizing well-being: The empirical encounter of two traditions. *Journal of Personality and Social Psychology* 82:1007–1022.

Keyes, K. M., B. F. Grant, D. S. Hasin. 2008. Evidence for a closing gender gap in alcohol use, abuse, and dependence in the United States population. *Drug and Alcohol Dependence* 11:21–29.

Khantzian, E. 1999. *Treating addiction as a human process*. Northvale, NJ: Jason Aronson.

Khantzian, E. J., J. E. Mack. 1994. How AA works and why it's important for clinicians to understand. *Journal of Substance Abuse Treatment* 11: 77–92.

Kiefer, F., H. Helwig, T. Tarnaske, C. Otte, H. Jahn, K. Wiedermann. 2005. Pharmacological relapse prevention of alcoholism: Clinical predictors of outcome. *European Addiction Research* 11: 83–91.

Klein, S., S. Lehmann. 2006. The science of happiness: *How our brains make us happy—and what we can do to get happier*. New York: Avalon.

Kling, M. A., R. E. Carson, L. Borg, A. Zametkin, J. A. Matochik, J. Schluger, P. Herscovitch, K. C. Rice, A. Ho, W. C. Eckelman, et al. (2000). Opioid receptor imaging with PET and [18F] cyclofoxy in long-term methodone-treated former heroin addicts. *Journal of Pharmacological and Experimental Therapeutics* 295 (3): 1070–1076.

Kluger, M. T., T. M. Laidlaw, N. Kruger, M. J. Harrison. 1999. Personality traits of anaesthetists and physicians: An evaluation using the Cloninger Temperament and Character Inventory (TCI-125). *Anaesthesia* 54 (10): 926–935.

Koenig, H.G. et. al. (2000) Handbook of religion and health. N.Y. Oxford University Press.

Koesters, M., T. Becker, R. Kilian, J. M. Fegert, S. Weinmann. 2009. Limits of meta-analysis: Methylphenidate in the treatment of adult attention-deficit hyperactivity disorder. *Journal of Psychopharmacology* 23 (7): 733–744.

# References

Kohut, H. 1971. The analysis of the self: *A systematic approach to the psychoanalytic treatment of narcissistic personality disorders*. Chicago: University of Chicago Press.

Kolla, B. P., M. P. Mansukhani, T. Schneekolth. 2011. Pharmacological treatment of insomnia in alcohol recovery: A systematic review. *Alcohol and Alcoholism*, 46 (5): 578–585.

Koob, G. F. 2000. Neurobiology of addiction: Toward the development of new therapies. *Annals of the New York Academy of Sciences* 909: 170–185.

Koob, G. F., M. J. Kreek. 2007. Stress, dysregulation of drug reward pathways and the transition to drug dependence. *American Journal of Psychiatry*, 164: 1149–1159.

Koob, G. F., M. LeMoal. 2001. Drug addiction dysregulation of reward and allostatis. *Neuropsychopharmacology* 24: 97–129.

Kosten, T. R., T. P. George. 2002. The neurobiology of opioid dependence: Implications for treatment. *Science and Practice Perspectives* (July): 13–21.

Kubler-Ross, E. 1969. *On death and dying*. New York: Macmillan.

Kurtz, E. 1979. Not-God: A history of Alcoholics Anonymous: Center City, MN: Hazelden Pittman Archives Press.

Kurtz, E., and K. Ketcham. 1992. *The spirituality of imperfection*. New York: Bantam Books.

Largman, R. 2009. Ignite the flame of intention. *Science of Spirituality*, http://empireofhope.wordpress.com

Laundergan, J. C. 1982. *Easy does it: Alcoholism treatment outcomes, Hazelden, and the Minnesota Model*. Center City, MN: Hazelden.

Leavitt, M. 2008. *Physical activity guidelines for Americans*. October, ODPHP Publication No. U0036. Secretary of the Department of Health and Human Services.

LeBon, O., P. Basiaux, E. Steel, J. Tecco, P. Minner, I. Pelc, P. Verbanck, S. Dupont. (2004). Personality profile and drug of choice: A multivariate analysis using Cloninger's TCI on heroin addicts, alcoholics, and a random population group. *Drug and Alcohol Dependence*, 73:175–182.

Leshner, A. 1997. Addiction is a brain disease, and it matters. *Science* 278 (October 3): 45–47.

Linley, P. A., and S. Joseph. 2004. Positive psychology in practice. Hoboken, NJ: John Wiley & Sons.

Lion, L. S. 1978. Psychological effects of jogging: A preliminary study. *Perceptual and Motor Skills* 47:1215–1218.

Lopez, S. 2009. Encyclopedia of positive psychology. Malden, MA: Wiley-Blackwell.

Lukasiewicz, M., X. Neveu, L. Blecha, B. Falissard, M. Reynaud, I. Gasquet. 2008. Pathways to substance-related disorder: A structural model approach exploring the influence of temperament, character, and childhood adversity in a national cohort of prisoners. *Alcohol and Alcoholism* 43 (3): 287–295.

Lykken, D. 1999. *Happiness: What studies on twins show us about nature, nurture, and the happiness set point.* New York: Golden Books.

Lynksey, M. T., and W. Hall. 2001. Attention deficit hyperactivity disorder and substance use disorders: Is there a causal link? *Addiction* 96 (6): 815–822.

Lyubormirsky, S. 2008. *The how of happiness: A scientific approach to getting the life you want.* New York: Penguin Press.

Mack, J. E. 1981. Alcoholism, AA, and the governance of the self. In *Dynamic Approaches to the Understanding and Treatment of Alcoholism*, edited by M. H. Bean and N. E. Zinberg. New York: Free Press, 128–162.

Mahesh Yogi, M. 1963. *The science of being and art of living: Transcendental Meditation.* New York: Allied.

Martinotti, G., C. R. Cloninger, L. Janiri. 2008. Temperament and Character Inventory dimensions and anhedonia in detoxified substance-dependent subjects. *The American Journal of Drug and Alcohol Abuse* 34 (2): 177–183.

Marura, S., A. B. Laudet, D. Mahmood, A. Rosenblum, H. S. Vogal, E. L. Knight. 2003. Role of self-help processes in achieving abstinence among dually diagnosed persons. *Addictive Behaviors* 3 (28): 399–413c.

Masse, L. C., and R. E. Tremblay. 1997. Behavior of boys in kindergarten and the onset of substance abuse during adolescence. *Archives of General Psychiatry* 54: 62–68.

Maxwell, M. A. 1984. *The Alcoholics Anonymous experience: A close-up view for professionals.* New York: McGraw-Hill.

# References

Mayter, G. S., K. J. Scott. 1988. An exploration of heterogeneity in an inpatient male alcoholic population. *Journal of Personality Disorders* 2:243–255.

McClernon, F. J., W. S. Yancy, J. A. Eberstein, R. C. Atkins, E. C. Westman. 2007. The effects of a low-carbohydrate ketogenic diet and a low-fat diet on mood, hunger, and other self-reported symptoms. *Obesity* 15 (1): 182–187.

McElrath, D. 1997. The Minnesota Model. *Journal of Psychoactive Drugs* 29:141–144.

McGee, M. 2008. Meditation and psychiatry. *Psychiatry* 5:28–41.

McGovern, M. P., D. H. Angres, M. Shaw, P. Rawal. 2003. Gender of physicians with substance use disorders: Clinical characteristics, treatment utilization, and post-treatment functioning. *Substance Use and Misuse* 38 (7): 993–1001.

McGovern, M. P., D. H. Angres, N. D. Uziel-Miller, S. Leon. 1998. Female physicians and substance abuse: Comparisons with male physicians presenting for assessment. *Journal of Substance Abuse Treatment* 15: 525–533.

McGovern, T., W. White, eds. 2002. *Alcohol problems in the United States.* New York: The Haworth Press.

McKellar, J., E. Stewart, K. Humphreys. 2003. Alcoholics Anonymous involvement and positive alcohol-related outcomes. *Journal of Consulting and Clinical Psychology* 2 (71): 302–308.

McLellan, A. T., D. Lewis, C. O'Brien, H. Kleber, H. 2000. Drug dependence, a chronic medical illness: Implications for treatment, insurance, and outcomes evaluation. *Journal of the American Medical Association* 284 (13): 1689–1695.

McLellan, A. T., G. S. Skipper, M. Campbell, R. L. DuPont. 2008. Five-year outcomes in a cohort study of physicians treated for substance use disorders in the United States. *British Medical Journal,* 337:a2038.

Miller, F. T. 1994. Protracted alcohol withdrawal delirium. *Journal of Substance Abuse Treatment* 11 (2): 127–130.

Miller, M., T. Gorski, D. Miller. 1982. Learning to live again: A guide for recovery from chemical dependency (revised). Independence, MO: Independence Press.

Miller, W., ed. 2000. *Integrating spirituality into treatment: Resources for practitioners.* Washington, D.C.: American Psychological Association.

Millon, T. 1997. *MCMI-III manual*. Minneapolis, MN: National Computer Systems.

Millon, T., S. Grossman, C. Millon, S. Meagher, R. Ramnath. 2004. Personality disorders in modern life, 2nd edition.. Hoboken, NJ: John Wiley & Sons.

Minnesota Recovery Page. 2009. Dry drunk syndrome. www.minnesotarecovery.info/literature/dry-drunk.htm.

Mishra, B. R., S. H. Nizamie, B. Das, S. K. Praharaj. 2009. Efficacy of repetitive transcranial magnetic stimulation in alcohol dependence: A sham-controlled study. *Addiction* 105:49–55.

Morgenstern, J., C. Kahler, R. Frey, E. Labouvie. 1996. Modeling therapeutic response to 12-step treatment: Optimal responders, non-responders, and partial responders. *Journal of Substance Abuse* 1 (8): 45–59.

Morral, A., M. Reti, D. McCaffrey, G. Ridgeway. 2001. Phoenix Academy treatment outcomes: Preliminary findings from the adolescent outcomes study. *NIDA Research Monograph* 182:111–112.

Morse, R. M., D. K. Flavin. 1992. The definition of alcoholism. *Journal of the American Medical Association* 268 (8): 1012–1014.

Nace, E. 2003. The importance of Alcoholics Anonymous in changing destructive behavior. *Primary Psychiatry* 10 (9): 65–72.

Najavits, L. M., P. Crits-Christoph, A. Dierberger. 2000. Clinicians' impact on the quality of substance use disorder treatment. *Substance Use and Misuse* 35 (12–14): 2161–2190.

National Council on Alcoholism and Drug Dependence. 2011. Alcoholism and alcohol-related problems: Fact sheet. New York: National Council on Alcoholism and Drug Dependence, www.ncadd.org.

National Institute on Alcohol Abuse and Alcoholism. 2003. The genetics of alcoholism. *Alcohol Alert* 60, 1–5, http://pubs.niaaa.nih.gov/publications/aa60.htm.

National Institute on Drug Abuse. 2002. Therapeutic community. *NIDA Research Report Series*, 1–12.

Neff, J. A., and S. A. MacMaster. 2005. Spiritual mechanisms underlying substance abuse behavior change in faith-based substance abuse treatment. *Journal of Social Work Practice in the Addictions* 5 (3): 33–54.

Nettle, D. 2005. *Happiness: The science behind your smile*. New York: Oxford Press.

Newberg, A., and M. R. Waldman. 2010. *How God changes your brain: Breakthrough findings from a leading neuroscientist.* New York: Ballantine Books.

Newton, T. F., R. De La Garza, A. D. Kalechstein, D. Tziortzis, C. A. Jacobsen. 2009. Theories of addiction: Methamphetamine users' explanations for continuing drug use and relapse. *The American Journal on Addictions* 18:294–300.

Nielsen, P., S. Rojskjaer, M. Hesse. 2007. Personality-guided treatment for alcohol dependence: A quasi-randomized experiment. *The American Journal on Addictions* 16:357–364.

Noel, X., M. Van Der Linden, A. Bechara. 2006. The neurocognitive mechanisms of decision-making, impulse control, and loss of willpower to resist drugs. *Psychiatry* 3 (5): 30–41.

Norwood, R. 1986. *Women who love too much: When you keep wishing and hoping he'll change.* New York: Pocket Books.

Ohlmeier, M. D., K. Peters, B. T. Te Wildt, M. Zedler, M. Ziegenbein, B. Wiese, H. M. Emrich, U. Schneider. 2008. Comorbidity of alcohol and substance dependence with attention-deficit/hyperactivity disorder (ADHD). *Alcohol and Alcoholism* 43 (3): 300–304.

Olds, J. 1956. Pleasure centers in the brain. *Scientific American*, 195: 105–116.

O'Malley, S. S., and J. C. Froehlich. 2002. Advances in the use of naltrexone: An integration of preclinical and clinical findings. *Recent Developments in Alcoholism* 16 (4): 217–245.

Ong, A. D., and M. H. M. van Dulmen. 2007. *Oxford handbook of methods in positive psychology.* New York: Oxford University Press.

Palmer, R. H. C., S. E. Young, C. J. Hopfer, R. P. Corley, M. C. Stallings, T. J. Crowley, J. K. Hewitt. 2009. Developmental epidemiology of drug use and abuse in adolescence and young adulthood: Evidence of generalized risk. *Drug and Alcohol Dependence* 102:78-87.

Parsian, A., C. R. Cloninger. 1997. Human GABA receptor alpha 1 and alpha 3 subunits genes and alcoholism. *Alcoholism Clinical and Experimental Research* 21 (3): 430–433.

Parsian, A., C. R. Cloninger, Z. H. Zhang. 2000. Functional variant in the DRD2 receptor promoter region and subtypes of alcoholism. *American Journal of Medical Genetics* 96 (3): 407–411.

Pearson, O. 2010. Anger and alcohol abuse. Livestrong, May 24. www.livestrong.com/article/130023-anger-alcohol-abuse/

Peniston, E.G., D. A. Marrinan, W. A. Deming, P. J. Kulkosky. 1993. EEG alpha-theta brainwave synchronization in Vietnam theater veterans with combat-related post-traumatic stress disorder and alcohol abuse. *Advances in Medical Psychotherapy* 6:37–50.

Peniston, E. G., and P. J. Kulkosky. 1989. Alpha-theta brainwave training and beta-endorphin levels in alcoholics. *Alcoholism: Clinical and Experimental Research* 13 (2): 271–277.

———. 1990. Alcoholic personality and alpha-theta brainwave training. *Medical Psychotherapy* 3:37–55.

Piderman, K. M., T. D. Schneekloth, V. S. Pankratz, S. D. Maloney, S. I. Altchuler. 2007. Spirituality in alcoholics during treatment. *The American Journal on Addictions* 16:232–237.

Potter-Efron, R., and P. Potter-Efron. 1995. Letting go of anger: The 10 most common anger styles and what to do about them. Oakland, CA: New Harbinger Publications, Inc.

Prochaska, J. O., and L. L. DiClemente. 1982. Transtheoretical therapy: Toward a more integrated model of change. *Psychotherapy* 19:276–288.

Project Match Research Group. 1997. Matching alcoholism treatments to client heterogeneity: Project Match posttreatment drinking outcomes. *Journal of Addictive Studies in Alcohol* 58:7–29.

Prosser, G., P. Carson, R. Phillips, A. Gelson, N. Buch, H. Tucker, M. Neophytou, M. Lloyd, T. Simpson. 1981. Morale in coronary patients following an exercise programme. *Journal of Psychosomatic Research* 25 (6): 587–593.

Putnam, S. C. 2001. *Nature's Ritalin for the marathon mind: Nurturing your ADHD child with exercise.* Hinesburg, VT: Upper Access.

Raglin, J. S., and W. P. Morgan. 1987. Influence of exercise and quiet rest on state anxiety and blood pressure. *Medicine and Science in Sports and Science,* 19 (5): 456–463.

Rando, K., K. I. Hong., Z. Bhagwagar, C. S. Ray Li, K. Bergquist, J. Guarnaccia, R. Sinha. 2011. Association of frontal and posterior cortical gray matter volume with time to alcohol relapse: A prospective study. *American Journal of Psychiatry* 168:183–192.

Rawson, R., C. Cooper, C. Domier. n.d.. Exercise as a novel approach to treat substance use disorders. In preparation.

Reilly, P. M., and M. S. Shopshire. 2002. Anger management for substance abuse and mental health clients: A cognitive behavioral therapy manual. DHHS Pub. No. (SMA) 02-3661. Rockville,

# References

MD: Center for Substance Abuse Treatment, Substance Abuse and Mental Health Services Administration.

Robbins, J. 2000. *A symphony in the brain.* New York: Grove Press.

Robins, Lee N. 1973. *The Vietnam drug user returns.* Washington, D.C.: U.S. Government Printing Office.

Rosario, T. 1987. An investigation of heterogeneity through personality assessment in a male inpatient alcoholic population. *Dissertations from ProQuest.* Paper 2625. http://scholarlyrepository.miami.edu/dissertations/2625.

Rounsaville, B. J., H. R. Kranzler, S. Ball, H. Tennen, J. Poling, E. Triffleman. 1998. Personality disorders in substance abusers: Relation to substance use. *Journal of Nervous and Mental Disease* 186:87–95.

Ryan, R. M., E. L. Deci. 2001. On happiness and human potentials: A review of research on hedonic and eudaimonic well-being. *Annual Review of Psychology* 52:141–166.

Rychlak, J. F. 1969. Lockean vs. Kantian theoretical models and the "cause" of therapeutic change. *Psychotherapy: Theory, Research, and Practice* 6:214–223.

Ryff, C. D., B. H. Singer, G. Dienberg Love. 2004. Positive health: Connecting well-being with biology. *Philosophical Transactions of the Royal Society of London,* 359:1383–1394.

Ryff, C. D., C. L. Keyes. 1995. The structure of psychological well-being revisited. *Journal of Personality and Social Psychology* 69:719–727.

SAMHSA. 2006. Results from the 2005 National Survey on Drug Use and Health: National findings. Rockville, MD: Office of Applied Studies, NSDUH Series H-30, DHHS Publication No. SMA 06-494.

SAMHSA. 2007. Most who need addiction treatment don't receive it. *American Society of Addiction Medicine Newsletter* 22 (Fall): 3, www.asam.org.

Sandoz, J. 2004. *Exploring the spiritual experience in the 12-step program of Alcoholics Anonymous. Spiritus contra spiritum.* Lewiston, NY: Edwin Mellon Press.

Scheff, L., and S. Edmiston. 2010. *The cow in the parking lot: A Zen approach to overcoming anger.* New York: Workman Publishing Company, Inc.

Scheff, T. J. 1974. The labeling theory of mental illness. *American Sociological Review*, 39:444–452.

Schore, A. N. 1994. *Affect regulation and the origin of the self: The neurobiology of emotional development.* Hillsdale, NJ: Lawrence Erlbaum Associates, Inc.

Schulman, M. 2002. How we become moral: The sources of moral motivation. In *Handbook of Positive Psychology*, edited by C. R. Snyder & S. J. Lopez, 499–514). New York: Oxford University Press.

Schwartz, J. M., and S. Begley. 2002. *The mind and the brain: Neuroplasticity and the power of mental force.* New York: Harper Collins.

Seeman, T. E. 1996. Social ties and health: The benefits of social integration. *Annals of Epidemiology* 6 (5): 442–451.

Segal, Z. V., J. M. Williams, J. D. Teasdale. 2002. *Mindfulness-based cognitive therapy for depression: A new approach to preventing relapse.* New York: The Guilford Press.

Seligman, M. E. P. 1995. The effectiveness of psychotherapy: The *Consumer Reports* study. *American Psychologist* 50:965–974.

———. 2002. *Authentic happiness: Using the new positive psychology to realize your potential for lasting fulfillment.* New York: Free Press.

———. 2011. Flourish. New York: Free Press

Sevarino, K. A., and T. R. Kosten. 2009. Naltrexone for initiation and maintenance of opiate abstinence. *Contemporary Neuroscience* 3:227–245.

Shermer, M. 2004. *The science of good and evil: Why people cheat, gossip, care, share, and follow the Golden Rule.* New York: Henry Holt & Company, LLC.

Siegel, D. J. 1999. *The developing mind: How relationships and the brain interact to shape who we are.* New York: The Guilford Press.

———. 2007. *The mindful brain: Reflection and attunement in the cultivation of well-being.* New York: W. W. Norton & Company.

Silverman, S. M. 2009. Opioid-induced hyperalgesia: Clinical implications for the pain practitioner. *Pain Physician* 12:679–684.

# References

Skeel, R. L., C. Pilarshi, K. Pytlak, J. Neudecker. 2008. Personality and performance-based measures in the prediction of alcohol use. *Psychology of Addictive Behaviors* 22 (3): 402–409.

Skodol, A. E., J. M. Oldham, P. E. Gallaher. 1999. Axis II comorbidity of substance use disorders among patients referred for treatment of personality disorders. *The American Journal of Psychiatry* 156 (5): 733–738.

Slotema, C. W., J. D. Blom, H. W. Hoek, I. E. C. Sommer. 2010. Should we expand the toolbox of psychiatric treatment methods to include repetitive Transcranial Magnetic Stimulation (rTMS)? A meta-analysis of the efficacy of rTMS in psychiatric disorders. *Journal of Clinical Psychiatry* 71 (7): 873–884.

Smith, M., G. Glass, T. Miller. 1980. *The benefit of psychotherapy*. Baltimore, MD: Johns Hopkins University Press.

Smits, J. A. J., A. C. Berry, D. Rosenfield, M. B. Powers, E. Behar, M. W. Otto. 2008. Reducing anxiety sensitivity with exercise. *Depression and Anxiety* 25 (8): 689–699.

Snyder, C. R., Lopez, S. J. (Eds.) (2002, 2009). Handbook of positive psychology. New York: Oxford University Press.

So, H.W. (2005). Substance abuse and psychiatric comorbidity: Millon Clinical Multiaxial Inventory III profiles of Chinese substance abusers. *Hong Kong Journal of Psychiatry* 15:89–96.

Spielberger, C. D., S. S. Krasnker, and E. P. Soloman. 1988. The experience, expression, and control of anger. In *Health psychology: individual differences and stress*, edited by M. P. Janisse, 89–108. New York: Springer.

Spicer, J. 1993. *The Minnesota Model: The evolution of the multidisciplinary approach to addiction recovery*. Center City, MN: Hazelden Educational Materials.

Staines, G., S. Magura, A. Rosenblum, C. Fong, N. Kosanke, J. Foote, A. Deluca. 2003. Predictors of drinking outcomes among alcoholics. *American Journal of Drug and Alcohol Abuse* 1 (29): 203–218.

Stanley, B., and L. J. Siever. 2010. The interpersonal dimension of borderline personality disorder: Toward a neuropeptide model. *American Journal of Psychiatry* 167:24–39.

Svrakic, D. M., C. Whitehead, T. R. Przybeck, C. R. Cloninger. 1993. Differential diagnosis of personality disorders by the seven-factor model of temperament and character. *Archives of General Psychiatry* 50:991–999.

Svrakic, D. M., S. Draganic, K. Hill, C. Bayon, T. R. Przybeck, C. R. Cloninger. 2002. Temperament, character, and personality disorders: Etiologic, diagnostic, treatment issues. *Acta Psychiatrica Scandinavica* 106 (3): 189–195.

Swendsen, J. D., K. P. Conway, B. J. Rounsaville, K. R. Merikangas. 2002. Are personality traits familial risk factors for substance use disorders? Results of a controlled family study. *The American Journal of Psychiatry* 159 (10): 1760–1766.

Swift, R. M. 2002. Drug therapy for alcohol dependence. *Treatment of substance use disorders*, edited by K. A. Sevarino, 35–54. New York: Brunner-Routledge.

Taylor, A. H., M. H. Ussher, G. Faulkner. 2007. The acute effects of exercise on cigarette cravings, withdrawal symptoms, affect, and smoking behaviour: A systematic review. *Addiction* 102:534–543.

Thanos, P. K., A. Tucci, J. Stamos, L. Robison, G. J. Wang, B. J. Anderson, N. D. Volkow. 2010. Chronic forced exercise during adolescence decreases cocaine conditioned place preference in Lewis rats. *Behavioral Brain Research* 215:77–82.

Tellegen, A., and N. G. Waller. 1987. Reexamining basic dimensions of natural language trait descriptors. Paper presented at the 95th annual convention of the American Psychological Association.

Terracciano, A., C. E. Lockenhoff, R. M. Crum, J. Bienvenu, P. T. Costa. 2008. Five-factor model personality profiles of drug users. *BMC Psychiatry* 8: 22.

Tolle, E. 1999. *Practicing the power of now: Essential teachings, meditations, and exercises from the power of now*. Novato, CA: New World Library.

———. 2003. *Stillness speaks*. Novato, CA: New World Library.

———. 2006. *A new Earth: Awakening your life's purpose*. New York: Plume Penguin.

Trivedi, M. H., T. L. Greer, B. D. Grannemann, H. O. Chambliss, A. N. Jordan. 2006. Exercise as an augmentation strategy for treatment of major depression. *Journal of Psychiatric Practice* 12 (4): 205–213.

United States Department of Agriculture. 2011. The Food Guide Pyramid. http://www.nal.usda.gov/fnic/Fpyr/pmap.htm

Vaillant, G. E. 1992. *Ego mechanisms of defense: A guide for clinicians and researchers*. Washington, D.C.: American Psychiatric Press.

Van den Heuvel, M. P., R. C. W. Mandl, R. S. Kahn, H. E. Hulshoff Pol. 2009. Functionally linked resting-state networks reflect the underlying structural connectivity architecture of the human brain. *Human Brain Mapping* 30:3127–3144.

Van den Wildenberg, E., R. W. Wiers, J. Dessers, R. G. Janssen, E. H. Lambrichs, H. J. Smeets, G. J. van Breukelen. 2007. A functional polymorphism of the mu-opioid receptor gene (OPRM1) influences cue-induced craving for alcohol in male heavy drinkers. *Alcohol Clinical and Experimental Research* 31 (1): 1–10.

Van Der Kolk, B. A. 2006. Clinical implications of neuroscience research in PTSD. *Annals of the New York Academy of Sciences,* 1071: 277–293.

Vanem, P., D. Krog, E. Hartmann. 2008. Assessment of substance abusers on the MCMI-III and the Rorschach. *Scandinavian Journal of Psychology* 49:83–91.

Van Wormer, K., and D. R. Davis. 2008. *Addiction treatment: A strengths perspective*, 2nd ed. Belmont, CA: Thomson Brooks/Cole.

Verheul, R., W. van den Brink, C. Hartgers. 1995. Prevalence of personality disorders among alcoholics and drug addicts: an overview. *European Addiction Research* 1:166–177.

Verheul, R., W. van den Brink, P. Geerlings. 1999. A Three-pathway psychobiological model of craving for alcohol. *Alcohol and Alcoholism* 34 (2): 197–222.

Vogel, R. A., P. T. Lehr. 2008. *The Pritikin edge: 10 essential ingredients for a long and delicious life.* New York: Simon & Schuster.

Wallace, A. B. 2006. *The attention revolution: Unlocking the power of the focused mind.* Boston: Wisdom Publications.

———. 2007. *Contemplative science: Where Buddhism and neuroscience converge.* New York: Columbia University Press.

Watkins, T., A. Lewellen, M. Barrett. 2001. *Dual diagnosis: An integrated approach to treatment.* Thousand Oaks, CA: Sage Publications.

W, Bill. 1976. *Alcoholics Anonymous: The story of how many thousands of men and women have recovered from alcoholism.* New York: Alcoholics Anonymous World Services.

Wegscheider-Cruse, S. 1985. *Choice-making for co-dependents, adult children, and spirituality seekers.* Pompano, FL: Health Communications.

Welwood, J., ed. 1992. *Ordinary magic: Everyday life as spiritual path*. Boston: Shambhala Publications.

White, W. 1998. *Slaying the dragon*. Bloomington, IL: Chestnut Health Systems.

Wiederman, M. 2007. Why it's so hard to be happy. *Scientific American Mind*, February/March:36–43.

Williamson, G. M., and M. S. Clark. 1989. Effects of providing help to another and of relationship type on the provider's mood and self-evaluation. *Journal of Personality and Social Psychology* 56:722–734.

Wills, T. A., D. Vaccaro, G. McNamara. 1994. Novelty seeking, risk taking, and related constructs as predictors of adolescent substance use: An application of Cloninger's theory. *Journal of Substance Abuse* 6:1–20.

Wolf, M. E. 2003. LTP may trigger addiction. *Molecular Interventions* 3 (5): 248–252.

World Health Organization. 2010. *ATLAS on substance use (2010): Resources for the prevention and treatment of substance use disorders*. Geneva, Switzerland: WHO Press.

Zanarini, M. C., F. R. Frankenburg, E. D. Dubo, A. E. Sickel, A. Trikha, A. Levin, V. Reynolds. 1998. Axis I comorbidity of borderline personality disorder. *American Journal of Psychiatry* 155:1733–1739.

Zimmerman, M., and W. Coryell. 1989. DSM-III personality disorder diagnoses in a nonpatient sample: Demographic correlates and comorbidity. *Archives of General Psychiatry* 46:682–689.

Zohar, D. 1991. *Quantum self*. New York: William Morrow and Company.

Zuckerman, M. 1994. *Behavioural expressions and biosocial bases of sensation seeking*. New York: Cambridge University Press.

9-4:00

Structured Living

Atena

Made in the USA
Lexington, KY
09 March 2015